CRASH COURSE
History and Physical Examination

History and
Physical
Examination

Paul R. Gordon, MD, MPH

Department of Family and Community Medicine
University of Arizona College of Medicine
Tucson, Arizona

UK edition authors
James Marsh and John Spencer

UK series editor
Wilf Yeo

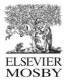

ELSEVIER
MOSBY

ELSEVIER
MOSBY

1600 John F. Kennedy Blvd.
Ste 1800
Philadelphia, PA 19103-2899

CRASH COURSE: HISTORY AND PHYSICAL EXAMINATION   ISBN 0-323-03561-2
Copyright 2005, Elsevier, Inc. All right reserved.

Notice

Knowledge and best practice in this field are constantly changing. As new research and experience broaden our knowledge, changes in practice, treatment and drug therapy may become necessary or appropriate. Readers are advised to check the most current information provided (i) on procedures featured or (ii) by the manufacturer of each product to be administered, to verify the recommended dose or formula, the method and duration of administration, and contraindications. It is the responsibility of the practitioner, relying on their own experience and knowledge of the patient, to make diagnoses, to determine dosages and the best treatment for each individual patient, and to take all appropriate safety precautions. To the fullest extent of the law, neither the Publisher nor the Author assumes any liability for any injury and/or damage to persons or property arising out or related to any use of the material contained in this book.

The Publisher

Previous edition copyrighted 1999, 2004.

Library of Congress Cataloging-in-Publication Data

Gordon, Paul.
    History and physical examination / Paul Gordon.—1st ed.
        p. ;   cm.—(Crash course)
    ISBN 0-323-03561-2
    1. Physical diagnosis.   2. Medical history taking.   I. Title.   II. Series.
    [DNLM: 1. Medical History Taking.   2. Physical Examination. WB 290 G664h 2005]
    RC76.G67 2005   2004063169
    616.07'51—dc22

Commissioning Editor: Alex Stibbe
Project Development Manager: Stan Ward
Project Manager: David Saltzberg
Designer: Andy Chapman
Cover Design: Richard Tibbets
Illustration Manager: Mick Ruddy

Printed in China

Last digit is the print number: 9   8   7   6   5   4   3   2   1

Preface

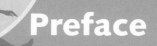

Crash Course: History and Physical Examination provides an integrated approach to the basic components of patient interactions: the medical history and the physical examination. The book begins each section with an overview. The student is introduced to the general medical interview and physical examination. Well suited for the student whose basic science curriculum follows a systems approach, the book then presents chapters on each of the body's systems, allowing the student to focus more closely on that system. For example, when taking a history of a patient with cardiovascular disease, the student is directed to more specific questions on that system. Similarly, the chapter about the physical examination of the cardiovascular system focuses on specific maneuvers relevant to that system. Each section uses specific clinical cases to direct the student's learning.

The content of *Crash Course: History and Physical Examination*, as noted above, makes it especially suitable for students in a systems approach to the basic sciences. Students during their clerkships who would like to review the basics and students who are beginning professional programs in the allied health sciences will also find this text helpful. Students studying in a more traditional basic sciences curriculum will also discover this text a useful tool for teaching them the history and physical exam and will determine the clinical cases to be stimulating. These cases will allow the student to integrate the various components of their basic sciences curriculum. This text will not serve as a detailed, in-depth reference source for topics in each of the clinical systems presented, but it is my hope that its integrated approach will allow students to incorporate the various components of their basic sciences curriculum as they proceed in their development as clinicians.

Paul Gordon, M.D., M.P.H.

Contents

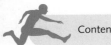

HISTORY TAKING

1. Introduction to the Medical Interview

Basic principles

The relationship between physician and patient is the cornerstone of medical care. One of the most important aspects of this relationship is the medical interview. Effective interviewers gather and evaluate data efficiently, demonstrate sensitivity to their patients' emotional needs, and determine acceptable treatments based on an understanding of the unique circumstances involved with each individual patient. Patients seek out and are more satisfied with clinicians who possess such interviewing skills. The goals of the medical interview are as follows:

Knowledge
- To understand how the use of the patient–doctor relationship can enhance communication and improve patient care.
- To understand the emotional effects of illness and how effective response to patient emotions affects diagnosis and treatment.

Skills
- To be able to interview a patient using the skills of the patient-centered medical interview listed in the interview checklist.
- Using these skills, students will be able to:
  - Elicit from patients their stories of illness, while pursuing the broader life setting in which symptoms occur.
  - Elicit from patients key information in their medical, family, and psychosocial histories.
  - Recognize and respond appropriately to a patient's emotions as they are expressed.
  - Support and encourage expression of patients' emotions.
  - Critically assess one's own performance and use of interviewing skill.
  - Develop interpersonal skills enabling the establishment of long-term relationships with patients.

Attitudes
- An unconditional positive regard for patients.
- A willingness to join patients as partners.
- A willingness to work with and learn from patients with diverse backgrounds and personal styles.

Patient-centered medical interview

Using patient-centered interviewing skills, you will be able to communicate effectively with your patients, while making your patients comfortable in their communication with you. The intent of the patient-centered medical interview is to encourage patients to offer information freely and honestly and to discuss those things that are of most concern to them. As a result of the interview and your competent use of the related skills, the patient should feel satisfied and comforted.

It is important to realize that the routine interview can also be therapeutic. Therapeutic goals of the patient interview include:
- Setting the patient at ease.
- Reducing patient anxiety and depression.
- Comforting and reassuring through the use of relationship skills and touch when appropriate.
- Enhancing feelings of personal control and helping patients cope by providing information and explanations about the causes of illness.
- Setting appropriate expectations for the doctor–patient relationship
- Strengthening the bond between doctor and patient.
- Enhancing the effectiveness of therapies through use of modeling, suggestion, confidence, optimism, praise, support, and encouragement.

Overall, use of patient-centered medical interviewing skills should allow you to elicit relevant medical and psychosocial data for use in the diagnosis, care, and treatment of your patient's illness while promoting a positive and therapeutic exchange between you and your patient.

The patient-centered interview has a three-part structure composed of opening, exploration of the problem, and closing. Each part of this structure has specific characteristics that allow you to

3

communicate with the patient in an interactive and facilitative way. The patient-centered interview follows two parallel frameworks: the illness framework and the disease framework (Fig. 1.1). Although there is overlap, attention to these two allows the clinician to deliver patient-centered care.

Opening

The opening of the interview consists of eight tasks that allow you to set the patient at ease, assess the patient's communication skills, choose a proper communication style, and initiate discussion. These include:

- Greeting: a verbal greeting ("Good afternoon"), shaking the patient's hand, and asking the patient, "How would you like to be addressed?"
- Introducing yourself by name.
- Attention to self-comfort: sitting in a relaxed fashion will permit the focusing of your attention on the patient and the interview.

- Attention to patient's comfort: ensuring that the patient is comfortable.
- Minimizing distractions: ensuring privacy and quiet.
- Asking the patient what his/her understanding of the interview is; for example, ask the patient: "So what you are saying is...."
- Calibration: assessing the patient's communication skills and selecting the appropriate approach to the interview.
- Invitation to speak: initiating discussion with an open question or statement ("How can I help you?").

However tempting, do not ignore throwaway comments from the patient. They often carry the key to the whole problem. Never be in a rush. Time invested in taking a good history pays dividends in the long term.

Exploration of the problem (information gathering)

Most of the time spent in a typical interview is used to explore problems and gather information from the patient. This part of the patient-centered medical interview provides the primary medium by which the physician can gather important illness-related and life-context information to use in forming hypotheses, prescribing treatments, and planning other action when caring for the patient. Skills/guideposts used in this phase of the interview include:

- Ask "What else?" to ascertain all major concerns.
- Determining with the patient the priorities of problems to be discussed.
- Establishing and maintaining a narrative thread: facilitating the patient's story of illness.
- Open-to-closed cone questioning: focus on and explore an area of inquiry, starting with an open question, and gradually use more directed questions to elicit all of the details of the illness/life context.
- Clarifying any unclear statements made by the patient.

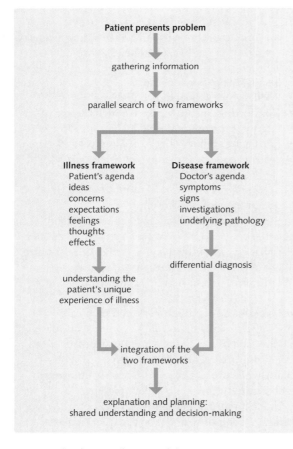

Fig. 1.1 The disease–illness model.

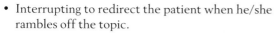

- Interrupting to redirect the patient when he/she rambles off the topic.
- Avoid asking more than one question at a time.
- Acknowledging the transition of the conversation from one topic area to another.

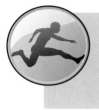

The history is the most important part of the patient's assessment as it provides 80% of the information required to make a diagnosis.

Closing

The closing of this part of the interview should include a summary of the patient's story and his/her feelings about an area of concern to the patient in order to check understanding and accuracy. It is also important to ask the patient if there is anything else he/she would like to discuss.

Physician as facilitator

In the patient-centered medical interview, the physician acts as facilitator, verbally and nonverbally encouraging the patient to tell his or her own story and share important information about him/her. You have several tools at your disposal that will help you in your role as facilitator:

- Eye contact: make eye contact with the patient. Sustain and repeat at comfortable intervals.
- Body positioning and body language: use open posture, arms uncrossed, facing the patient.
- Encouraging gestures (e.g., head nod).
- Nonverbal, vocal encouragement (e.g., "mm-hmm").
- Encouraging the patient to continue by repeating the last few words stated.
- Using silences to allow the patient to express his/her thoughts and feelings.
- Using relationship skills.

Responding to emotions and conveying empathy

Five relationship skills have been identified that can aid in your communication of empathy to patients. Relationship skills allow you to facilitate the patient's free expression of emotions and to support those emotions as they are expressed. Expression of empathy is one of the most potent of the physician's therapeutic interventions. Empathy is understanding another's emotions or feelings as if they are one's own. All people have a need to be understood, a need made more pressing by illness. Empathy involves accurately identifying a patient's feelings and then communicating this to the patient. In addition to strengthening the bond between doctor and patient, expression of empathy can aid the diagnostic process. After experiencing the physician's empathy, patients are often encouraged to reveal their most difficult problems. Communication of empathy can be accomplished through the use of skills that can be effectively learned. The five relationship skills used to respond to emotions and convey empathy include:

- Reflection: recognize and name emotions as they are expressed.
- Legitimation: express understandability of the patient's emotions.
- Respect: express respect for the patient's coping efforts.
- Support: express a willingness to be helpful to the patient in addressing his/her concerns.
- Partnership: express a willingness to work together with the patient to address concerns and solve problems.

Cultural awareness is a critically important aspect of our work as clinicians. The following questions (adapted from Kleinman) can assist us:

1. What do you call the problem?
2. What do you think has caused the problem?
3. Why do you think it started when it did?
4. What do you think this condition does? How does it work?
5. How severe is this condition? Will it have a short or long course?
6. What kind of treatment should you receive? What are the most important results you hope to receive from this treatment?

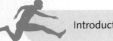

7. What are the chief problems the condition has caused?
8. What do you fear most about the condition?

The doctor–patient relationship has always been based on trust and respect. Interpersonal and communication skills are one of the core competencies as defined by the Accreditation Council for Graduate Medical Education (ACGME). The medical interview performed in a patient-centered model allows the physician to gain the trust and respect of the patient and help address this domain as defined by the ACGME.

2. The Medical Interview Framework: An Outline with Specific Questions

Key content of the interview

The interview should serve to provide key information to the physician. Key content areas covered in a patient-centered medical interview should include information about the patient's perception of and response to symptoms and the nature of home life and family relationships. The following content areas form the basis of the medical interview framework:
- Patient identification.
- Informant (patient or other) and reliability.
- Chief complaint.
- History of present illness.
- Past medical history.
- Family history.
- Social history.
- High-risk behaviors.
- Health maintenance and preventive care.
- Review of systems.

The collecting of information has always been viewed as the standard medical interview (Fig. 2.1). Indeed the information collected is critically important. However, knowing the right questions is only part of the medical interview. The way in which the questions are asked, the tone, body language, and relationship skills are all equally important. Without these skills, knowing the right questions will not result in the "right answers."

Throughout the interview, please remember the following principles:
- Introduce yourself and your role.
- Attend to the patient's comfort.
- Always begin with open-ended questions and allow the patient adequate time to answer (later narrowing to closed-cone, focused questions).
- Ask "What else?" to ascertain all major concerns.
- Avoid asking more than one question at a time.
- Use segment summaries: restate the content/feeling and check for accuracy.
- Use transitions.
- Use eye contact to enhance patient comfort.
- Maintain an open posture.

- Use a head nod, "mm-hmm," repeat the patient's last statement.
- Use silence to facilitate patient's expression of thoughts and feelings.
- Convey empathy using the skills of reflection, legitimization, respect, support, and partnership.
- Assess the patient's understanding of the disease/symptoms, etc.

Introduction

Introduce yourself to the patient and explain your role. Take this time to find out a little about your patient:
- Where are you from?
- What sort of work do/did you do?
- How did you choose the University Hospital for your care?

Identification

Name, age, gender, occupation, residence, referring and/or primary care physician.

Informant and reliability

If the reliability of the patient as a history giver is in doubt, a Folstein mini-mental status exam should be done here.

Chief complaint (CC)

The CC is a statement in the patient's own words of the index symptom that you have selected from the interview material as being chief or principal. Because it is a direct (albeit edited) quotation, it is placed in quotation marks.

History of present illness (HPI)

The present illness is not simply a disorganized catalog of statements and facts. The organization of this portion of the history is based on several principles:
- The major problem that the patient is suffering from must be dissected free of other unrelated information and developed in a chronological fashion.
- The major problem should be characterized by the use of the Sacred Seven:

Outline for normal adult interview

I. Introduction
1. Introduce self
2. Explain your role
3. Ask patient's name and age
4. Broad opening question

II. Chief complaint and history of present illness
1. Location/radiation
2. Timing
3. Quality
4. Severity
5. Setting or onset
6. Modifying factors
7. Associated symptoms

III. Past medical history
1. Childhood diseases, illnesses, hospitalizations, operations, accidents
2. Any other? Hospitalizations, operations, illnesses, accidents since childhood
3. Obtain documentation on pertinent items
4. Allergies
5. Treatments for specific problems
6. Current medications

IV. Family history
1. Immediate family
   a. Ages
   b. Current health
   c. Past health, accidents, etc.
   d. If dead, age and cause of death
   e. Chronic or hereditary diseases
   f. Be sensitive to patient's feelings regarding any death, or major illnesses
2. Other relatives (same as 1, a–f)

V. Social history
1. Marital status and previous marriages
2. Occupation of self and spouse or significant other
3. Children
4. Hobbies, other spare-time activities
5. Financial status (especially regarding healthcare)
6. Education
7. Community and religion
8. A typical day

VI. High-risk behaviors
1. Tobacco
2. Alcohol (consider using CAGE questions)
3. Recreational/illegal drugs
4. Do you use any prescription drugs in an abusive way (e.g., sleeping pills, pain pills)?
5. Eating disorder
6. Sexual history
7. Violence/abuse
8. Occupational hazards

VII. Health/preventive care
1. Sleep
2. Body weight/diet/caffeine
3. Exercise
4. Vaccinations
5. Injury prevention, seatbelts, helmets
6. Age-appropriate health screening activities

VIII. Review of systems
1. Be specific and complete
2. Use words that patients can understand

Fig. 2.1 Outline for normal adult interview.

1. Location/radiation: where is the pain or symptom and does it move
2. Timing: when did it begin; determine the rate of development of the symptom (Figs. 2.2 and 2.3).
3. Quality: ask the patient to describe it; if the patient cannot, offer options such as sharp, stabbing, dull, vice-like, burning, crushing, throbbing.
4. Severity: either use a visual analog scale or ask them to rate it from 1 to 10.
5. Setting or onset: what was the patient doing at the time it began.
6. Modifying factors: does anything make it better or worse.

7. Associated symptoms: these symptoms are often characteristic of certain pathological processes; they will be mentioned in subsequent chapters. Pertinent positives and negatives help clarify the major problem and demonstrate that you have given some thought to the differential diagnosis.

Past medical history (PMHx)

The PMHx allows you to identify risk factors that will help you arrive at a diagnosis.

• Current medications: name, dose, frequency, indications, starting date, include over-the-counter drugs and eye ointments, herbs, and dietary supplements.

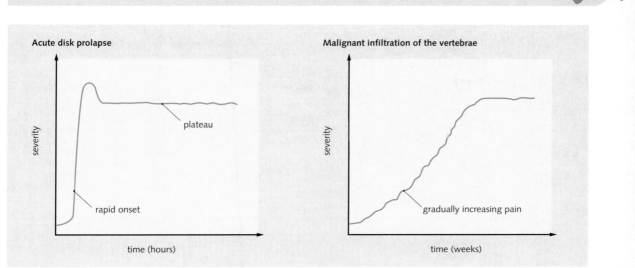

Fig. 2.2 Graphs illustrating the typical time course of two different types of back pain, which are of the same severity at presentation but of different etiology.

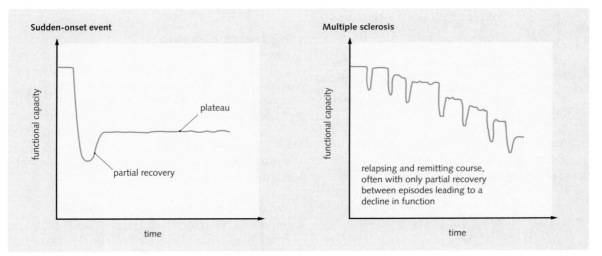

Fig. 2.3 Graph of the time course of functional capacity against time for a patient who has had a stroke or has multiple sclerosis. It is important to consider not only the speed of onset of a particular symptom but also its subsequent time course.

- Allergies/untoward reactions.
- Serious illness: record any serious infectious disease or prolonged illness.
- Injuries.
- Surgeries (hospitalized and outpatient): date, place, type, surgeon, complications.
- Childhood illnesses.
- Nonsurgical hospitalizations: date, place, doctor, reason, treatment, outcome.

Family history (FHx)

A family history identifies possible genetic risk factors and may help you understand the patient's current symptoms in the context of his/her family background.

- Include all first-degree relatives.
- Find out health status of all living first-degree relatives and their ages.

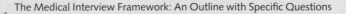

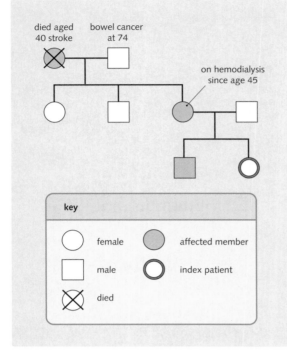

Fig. 2.4 A typical family tree written in hospital notes demonstrating family members affected by autosomal dominant polycystic kidneys.

- Find out how all deceased first-degree relatives died and at what age.
- A family pedigree is useful visually (Fig. 2.4).
- "Are there diseases that you think run in your family?" is a useful question that frequently uncovers what the patient fears he/she may have (Fig. 2.5).

Social history (SHx)

The social history will help you identify the context in which your patient is experiencing the illness. What support network do they have? Upon whom can they rely? Among cancer patients, research has demonstrated decreased morbidity with stronger social support networks. SHx includes:
- Birthplace.
- Hometown.
- Education.
- Work history.
- Marital status and adjustment.
- Significant others and where they are.
- Children, parents' occupations.

Examples of some inherited disorders	
Pattern of inheritance	**Examples**
autosomal dominant	adult-onset polycystic kidney disease; neurofibromatosis; familial adenomatous polyposis
autosomal recessive	cystic fibrosis; sickle-cell anemia; infantile polycystic kidney disease
X-linked recessive	color blindness; hemophilia A
X-linked dominant	vitamin D-resistant rickets

Fig. 2.5 Examples of some inherited disorders.

- Living circumstances.
- Outside interests.
- Daily activities.
- Financial status.

High-risk behaviors

Historically certain questions that have always been difficult to ask have fallen under the "Social History" section of the interview. I have chosen to make this a separate section of the interview, which we will call "high-risk behaviors." Furthermore, I have included a section with more detailed questions for selected behaviors at the end of this chapter. An asterisk (*) indicates the behaviors that have additional questions at the end of the chapter.

One should never choose to ask or not ask certain of these questions based on a "feeling or gut-level response." For example, this person does not do drugs or smoke, or this person is definitely gay or straight. Since "you can't tell a book by its cover" and these behaviors can result in significant health problems, all patients need to be asked.

Sensitive areas that require careful questioning include sexual history, risk factors for HIV infection, history of suicide/suicide attempts, history of family violence, and trauma screen.

By framing this section of the interview in the context of "certain behaviors can result in health problems and I want to assess your risks," it will be easier to ask your patients. In this section of the interview, you need to ask about the following high-risk behaviors:

Sex*
- Are you sexually active?
- Do you know about behaviors that may put you at risk for sexually transmitted diseases? (If the patient is uncertain or unclear, list those behaviors.)

Tobacco
- Do you use tobacco in any form?

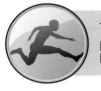

There are few diseases in adult patients for which a smoking history is not relevant.

Alcohol
- CAGE questions:
  - C = Have you ever felt you ought to Cut down on your drinking?
  - A = Have people Annoyed you by criticizing your drinking?
  - G = Have you ever felt bad or Guilty about your drinking?
  - E = Have you ever had a drink first thing in the morning to steady your nerves or get rid of a hangover—an Eye opener?
- A positive answer to two or more questions identifies the majority of people with alcohol abuse or dependence.

Recreational/illegal drugs
- Do you use any recreational or illegal drugs?
- Have you ever?
- If you used injectable drugs, have you ever shared needles?

Accidents
- Do you wear a seatbelt?
- Do you engage in any high-risk sports or activities?

Eating
- Are you satisfied with your eating patterns?
- Do you ever eat in secret?

Violence/abuse*
- Do you own guns?
- Have you ever been exposed to any emotional or physical violence?
- Have you ever been injured in an assault or fight?

Occupation
- Do you think you are exposed at work to any of the following:
  1. Unsafe conditions?
  2. Hazardous chemicals, solvents, or dusts?
  3. Other conditions you wish to discuss?

Health/preventive care
The two leading causes of death (heart disease and cancer) are linked to risk factors that are directly affected by lifestyle choices. This section of the interview gives you the opportunity to identify those areas.
- Sleep: ask patient to describe his/her sleep pattern.
- Body weight: loss/gain of >10lb; heaviest weight; what the patient considers a normal weight for him/herself.
- Exercise: frequency, type.
- Diet: estimated calories, % fat, fiber, sodium, calcium, iron, restrictions, advoidances.
- Date of last:
  1. Breast exam/mammogram.
  2. Pelvic/Pap exam.
  3. Prostate exam.
  4. Flexible sigmoidoscopy or colonoscopy.
  5. Cholesterol result.
  6. Testicular exam.
- Vaccinations: dT, pneumovax, influenza, hepatitis B, measles, rubella.
- Aspirin prophylaxis.
- Injury prevention: MVAs (seatbelts, alcohol/drugs, helmets), high risk for back, high risk for falls, fire safety, violence.
- Stress and bereavement.

Review of systems (ROS)
In the ROS you ask your patient a long list of questions to identify problems that the patient may have failed to mention. Many of these systems questions can be used in the HPI to help you gain

more detail about the patient's symptom. In subsequent chapters, many of these will be discussed in greater depth with clinical scenarios.

You will notice that only certain questions begin with "Have you ever had...." This introduction should be reserved for symptoms that are important to know about *whenever* they may have occurred. Avoid that introduction for every question. It should be rapidly clear that a question such as "Have you ever had a sore throat?" will (1) get a positive answer from every patient and (2) yield information of questionable relevance to understand a patient's *current* problem.

General
- Do you have fever?
- Any chills or sweats?
- Has your weight changed recently?
- Have you felt your health is "not up to par?"

Skin
- Do you have a skin problem?
- Do you have a skin rash?
- Do you itch?
- Any sores on your skin?
- Have you noticed any change in your hair or nails recently?

Hematopoietic system
- Do you have a tendency to bruising?
- Any bleeding from your gums?
- Have you ever bled excessively after an operation, dental procedure, or injury?
- Any history of anemia?

Head
- Are you bothered by severe headaches?
- Frequent headaches?
- Any history of head injury?

Eyes
- Do you have any problem with your eyes?
- How is your vision?
- Do you wear glasses or contacts?
- Do you ever see double?
- Do you ever see spots or flashes of light?
- Is there any pain in your eyes?

Ears
- Do you have any problems with your ears?
- How is your hearing?
- Do you have ringing or buzzing?
- Do you get dizzy?
- Any pain or discharge from the ears?

Nose
- Do you have nosebleeds?
- How is your sense of smell?
- Do you have any drainage from your nose?
- Does air pass freely through your nose?

Mouth
- What is the condition of your teeth?
- Any sore tongue?
- Are you troubled with sores in your mouth?

Pharynx and larynx
- How often do you have sore throats?
- Any hoarseness?

Neck
- Do you have any problem with your neck?
- Any swelling?
- Any swollen glands?

Respiratory system
- Do you have any trouble with your lungs?
- Do you have a cough?
- Do you cough anything up? (How much? What does it look like?)
- Have you ever coughed up blood?
- Are you short of breath?
- Do you wheeze?
- Do you have any pain anywhere in your chest?

Cardiovascular system
- Do you have a history of high blood pressure?
- Have you ever had a heart murmur?
- Do you have any chest discomfort? Where? Is it related to exertion? To breathing?
- Have you ever noticed fluttering or pounding of your heart?
- Do you have shortness of breath at night?
- Any swelling of your feet and ankles?
- Do you have pain in your calves while walking?
- Do you have varicose veins?
- Any history of phlebitis?

Gastrointestinal system
- Have you ever had trouble with your digestion or bowels?
- How is your appetite?

- Any trouble swallowing?
- Do you have heartburn or belching?
- Nausea?
- Vomiting?
- Have you ever vomited blood?
- Do you have pain anywhere in your abdomen?
- Have you ever turned yellow (been jaundiced)?
- How is your bowel function?
- Do you have pain with your bowel movements?
- Any trouble with hemorrhoids?

Urinary system
- Do you have kidney or bladder trouble?
- How often do you urinate in 24 hours?
- Any urination during the night?
- Do you have pain or burning on urination?
- Do you have trouble getting the stream started?
- Have you ever had blood in your urine?
- Any pain in your back?
- Do you ever lose control of your urine?

Genital system—female
- When did your menstrual periods begin?
- Have you ever been pregnant?
- How many living children?
- Any miscarriages?
- Do you have any problem with your periods?
- When was your last period?
- Do you use birth control measures?
- Have you ever had a venereal disease?
- Do you have any sexual problem?
- What is your sexual preference?
- Do you have a vaginal discharge?

Genital system—male
- Any history of sores on your genitals?
- Have you ever had a discharge from your penis?
- Any pain or swelling in your testicles?
- Have you ever had a venereal disease?
- Do you have any sexual problems?
- What is your sexual preference?

Endocrine system
- Any history of thyroid trouble?
- Goiter?
- Prominent eyes?
- Tremor?
- Have you ever had diabetes?
- Any history of excessive thirst?
- Markedly increased urine flow?

- Any change in your facial features, or in the size of your hands and feet?

Musculoskeletal system
- Do you have any trouble with your joints? Muscles?
- Any history of back trouble?
- Any pain in any of your joints? (Redness? Swelling?)
- Limitation of motion in a joint?
- Any history of injury to your bones or joints?

Neurological system
- Do you have any history of fainting? Loss of consciousness?
- Any history of convulsions or seizures?
- Have you noticed any recent change in memory?
- Have you ever been paralyzed?
- Has there been any loss of feeling anywhere?
- Do you have trouble with your coordination?
- Any trouble walking?
- Do you have any weakness of any of your muscles?

Psychiatric concerns
- Have you ever had any nervous or emotional problems?
- Have you ever had periods where you felt unusually depressed for days or weeks at a time?
- Any history of periods where you were unusually high-spirited for days or weeks at a time?
- Do you ever feel confused?
- Have you had trouble sleeping?
- Have you ever noticed thoughts that seemed strange or troubling to you?
- Have you noticed any change in your personality?
- Do you feel differently toward other people?

Responding to patient emotions

The second function of the interview concerns the development of rapport and responding to patient's emotions.

Objectives
- Develop and maintain rapport.
- Patient satisfaction: adherence and fewer lawsuits.
- Relief of distress.
- Detection and management of psychiatric illness.
- Physician satisfaction.
- Improved physical outcome.

Skills

- Reflection.
- Legitimization.
- Support.
- Partnership.
- Respect.

Many basic and higher-order skills can be used to improve doctor–patient rapport. However, the above five can serve as a core set of basic skills for this function.

Reflection

Recognize and name emotions as they are expressed. For example, "Mrs. Smith, I see this problem is disturbing to you," or "Mr. Jones, I realize that my keeping you waiting so long must be frustrating for you."

Legitimization

Refers to explicit statements by the physician that validate the patient's emotional response. For example, "I think anyone would find this information quite distressing."

Support

Express a willingness to be helpful to the patient in addressing his/her concerns. For example, "I am going to do whatever I can to help you overcome this problem."

Partnership

Express a willingness to work together with the patient to address concerns and solve problems. For example, "Let's talk about this problem and together try to develop some solutions."

Respect

Explicitly express recognition of the patient's accomplishments or coping efforts. For example, "I am impressed by the way you are handling your work and home life, in spite of the medical problems you've been having."

The delivering of bad news is a time when you will need to respond to a patient's emotions. Some of the principles to keep in mind when delivering bad news include the following:

- The physician's goal is to inform patient and family so that they are able to comprehend the clinical situation and make sound decisions consistent with their beliefs and ideals.

- Attend to the appropriateness of the surrounding; leave distractions (e.g., pager) elsewhere; sit in a quiet setting.
- Time the delivery to maximize the strength of all persons involved.
- If there is a language barrier, use an interpreter rather than a family member.
- Assess the patient's present physiological and emotional state.
- Prepare the patient by saying there is a difficult topic to discuss:

    Physician: Good morning. How are you feeling today?

    Patient: Better than I did a week ago.

    Physician: I'm glad of that. We have some very serious matters to discuss regarding your health. Do you feel ready for this discussion?

- Express sorrow for the patient's pain: be human.
- Give limited information; schedule time to talk again later.
- Be realistic; avoid the temptation to minimize the problem, but don't take away all hope.
- Explore how the patient feels after receiving the news.
- Reassure the patient of the continued availability of care no matter what happens.
- Physicians must be comfortable with uncertainty.

The difficult interview

It is never too early to learn skills that allow one to deal successfully with difficult patients. This is a common problem, and inability to deal with this group of patients is a common cause of professional dissatisfaction. The goal of this section is to enhance the interaction between the student and the difficult patient so that healthcare is optimized and the relationship is satisfying.

Objectives

- Identify the characteristics of a "difficult" patient.
- Recognize the "hidden agenda" within a patient's demands and behavior.
- Acknowledge your own negative feelings toward the patient's behavior.
- Acknowledge your own limitations.
- Acquire "tools" to manage these patients more effectively.
- Recognize responsibility in the management of these patients.

Skills
Practice the six-step approach:
- Recognize and acknowledge your feelings.
- Realize that you have a choice and may exercise it.
- Allow enough time.
- Ask: What is the patient really requesting?
- Ask: Am I able to help and to what extent?
- Ask: What else do I need? (i.e., resources).

More detailed questions for high-risk behaviors

At times, you might want more detailed questions while performing a high-risk behavior interview.

Sexual screen
- Are you sexually active at the present time?
- If no, have you ever been?
- Are (were) your partners men, women, or both?
- If both, which do you prefer?
- What means of birth control do you (have you) use(d)? Ask both males and females.
- Do you have any concerns or problems with your sexual life?
- Have there been any changes in your sexual activity?
- Changes in level and frequency of interest?
- Changes in type of interest?
- Do you engage or have you ever engaged in anal intercourse?
- Are there any ways in which you would like your sexual life to be different?
- Have any bad or frightening things ever happened to you sexually? For example: rape, sexual abuse, or molestation? (See Abuse Screen)
- Have you had any sexually transmitted diseases such as herpes, chlamydia, gonorrhea, syphilis, or AIDS? (See HIV Screen)
- Have you ever been treated for a sexually transmitted disease?

HIV risk factors
- Do you worry about getting AIDS? Why or why not?
- Do you practice safe sex? (Explain)
- Have you ever injected (or shot up) drugs into your veins?
- (If male) Have you ever had sexual contact with another man or with someone who used IV drugs?
- (If female) Have you ever had sexual contact with someone who was bisexual or someone who used IV drugs?
- How many sexual partners have you had in the last 10 years?
- Have you ever needed a blood transfusion? What year? (1979–1985 is risk period)

Suicide and violence screen
- Have you ever had thoughts that life is not worth living?
- Have you ever had thoughts of killing yourself? (Now?)
- How would you do it?
- Have you taken steps to carry out your plan? (e.g., collected weapons, pills)

Patients who are suicidal may also be homicidal and vice versa, so ask:
- Have you ever had thoughts of hurting anyone else? (Now?)
- Have you ever hurt anyone else?
- What plans do you now have to hurt anyone?

Screens for family violence
1. Child abuse (modify for male perpetrators)
- How did you feel during your pregnancy?
- Has your child lived up to your expectations?
- At what age do you think children know right from wrong? (Abusers often have unrealistically high expectations of children.)
- How do you feel when your child behaves badly? What do you do?
- Is there anyone you can turn to for help?
- Have you ever been concerned that anyone would hurt your child?
- Have you been frightened with thoughts of hurting your child?
- Have you or anyone else hurt your child?

2. Sexual abuse victims
- Are there things going on in your home that you are uncomfortable with or ashamed to talk about?
- Has there been any sexual contact between family members in your home besides your parents?
- Have you been involved sexually with any adult, including either of your parents?

3. Partner/elder abuse victims
- I know that you may be ashamed of what happened (or might have happened), but could it be that this injury did not happen by accident?

- Is your family under a lot of stress?
- What happens when you and your partner argue?
- Do either of you have trouble with your temper?
- Have you ever fought physically with your partner? How badly have you been hurt?
- Is there a weapon in the house?
- Are you afraid to go home?

4. Abuse history
- Did you ever witness any violence in your home when you were growing up?
- How were you disciplined as a child?
- Were you ever physically hurt by a family member?

During your childhood or adolescence:
- Did a relative, family friend, or stranger ever touch your body, or have you touch them, in a sexual way?

- Did anyone attempt or succeed in having sexual intercourse with you?
- Did you ever have an unwanted sexual experience of any kind?

Trauma screen
- Have you ever had anything happen to you where you thought you would be seriously injured or might die?
- Have you ever been in a life-threatening accident? Fire? Disaster?
- Have you ever been attacked or raped?
- Have you ever seen these things happen to someone else?

3. Interview of the Older Adult

Overview

The fastest-growing patient group in the twenty-first century is the older adult. This group of medical patients will feel empowered to take an active role in their own care. Older patients are concerned about slowing the effects of aging, maintaining health, managing chronic illness, and maximizing independence. Effective healthcare for older patients involves an awareness of their special needs. Physicians play a critical role and need the skills and knowledge to help guide and care for this population.

Objectives of geriatric interview

- Utilize techniques that foster respect and rapport.
- Identify biases that may interfere with the effective communication.
- Incorporate methods that enhance communication with the sensory impaired.
- Incorporate alternative sources of information.
- Address possible underreporting of illness.
- Efficiently collect information regarding function, medications, and nutrition.
- Increase awareness of disease states and altered presentation of illnesses.

Communication skills

- Reflection.
- Respect.
- Listening.
- Collaboration.
- Compassion (both verbal and nonverbal).

Reflection
Recognize how personal values and fears around aging may influence how one interacts and cares for older adults. For example, "Mrs. Lee, I often wonder how I will accept my own loss of independence and recognize that it must be frustrating."

Respect
Accept what is unique about each individual, including his/her personal strategies for adapting to the aging process. For example, "Mr. Lopez, I am glad to hear that your weekly acupuncture sessions are making you feel more energetic."

Listening
Allow patients to share things that are important in their lives along with their fears and concerns. For example, "Ms. Williams, thank you for sharing your story. I can see how important your family is to you."

Collaboration
Form a partnership with your patient as well as with other healthcare professionals. For example, "Mr. O'Connor, you and I are going to develop a plan with the physical therapist in order to restore strength in your legs."

Compassion (verbal)
Communicate your interest in the wellbeing of your patient. For example, "Mrs. Matsumoto, I want to take the time to hear how you're doing today."

Compassion (nonverbal)
Use appropriate touch, facial expressions, and/or body language, for example, the use of a genuine smile, pat on the back, or handshake. When in doubt, assess the comfort level by asking, for example, "Mrs. Bethel, is it okay to give you a hug?"

Principles for communicating with older adults

- The physician's goal is to develop communication techniques that address the biopsychosocial and spiritual needs of older adults.
- Attend to sensory losses that may complicate or slow down the communication process.
- Incorporate effective nonverbal techniques that reflect your caring and compassion.
- Recognize that aging alone is not a disease and that symptoms should not be attributed solely to growing old.

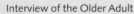

- Ask patients to share openly any new change in their health status because they often will underreport illnesses or attribute symptoms to aging.
- See the patient in the larger context of family, support system, and community.
- Be sensitive to the patient's relationship to the caregiver if one is present during the interview.
- Remember that the geriatric population is not a homogeneous population. Patients vary from the healthy and vital to the frail and dependent.
- Consider the individual's life experiences and how these may affect the perception of the healthcare system and the role of the physician.

Specific considerations in the history of the elderly patient

See Fig. 3.1.
- Attitudinal factors.
- Prejudice of ageism.
- Seeing patient as parent figure.
- Preconceived biases about elderly (rigid, easily angered, senile, dependent, unworthy, expendable, unimportant, useless).
- Allowing fear/resentment of one's own aging to affect relationships with elders (e.g., "What can you expect at your age?").
- Most older adults can meet the challenges of daily life with little or no assistance.
- Approximately 80% of persons aged 65 to 74 have no disability.
- Even after age 85, 40% of older persons remain fully functional.
- Failure to pursue "taboo" subjects.
- Sexuality: most older persons remain sexually active.
- Elder abuse: thought to affect at least 4% of elder population.

Communication difficulties
- Sensory losses may affect communication.
- Check if assistive devices (e.g., hearing aids, eyeglasses) are in place.
- Impaired hearing:
  - Do not presume that all elderly patients cannot hear.
  - Only 30% of persons over age 65 have hearing loss that affects everyday communications.
  - May lead to isolation and depression.

- Speak slowly and clearly.
- Face patient directly to facilitate lip-reading.
- Lean toward the patient.
- Eliminate distracting noises.
- Speak more loudly, but not higher-pitched.
- Supplement with written interview.
- Sign language is not too useful.

Do not presume that all elderly patients cannot hear. Only 30% of persons over age 65 have hearing loss that affects everyday communications.

- Impaired vision:
  - "It's so dark in here, I can't see anything."
  - Room should be well lit.
  - Minimize glare.
  - May not have good color vision.
- Dysarthria may be due to neurological problem or dentures.
- Aphasia: ask "yes–no" questions.
- Confusional state.

Mental status exam (if needed)
- Patient may recognize problem or deny.
- See at different times to fully assess.
- Some medical conditions and/or medications may cause confusion that mimics dementia.
- Dementia is not part of normal aging.
- Touching ("skin to skin") extremely useful even if unnecessary.

Establishing rapport/trust
- Sit when speaking.
- Use last name unless permission is granted otherwise.
- Begin with an explanation of what is to be accomplished.
- Utilize caring gestures when appropriate (handshake, pat on the back, shoulder touch).
- Eliminate physical barriers (such as furniture) between yourself and the patient.
- Minimize distractions and interruptions.
- Maintain eye contact when culturally appropriate.
- Communicate your concern and willingness to help.

Specific considerations in the history of the elderly patient

Attitudinal factors
Ageism, preconceived biases
Elders as parental figure
One's own aging
Expectations of advanced age
Failure to pursue taboo subjects
  (sexuality, abuse)

Communication difficulties
Sensory losses
Utilize assistive devices
Impaired hearing
Don't presume all cannot hear
Speak slowly and clearly
Face patient directly
Lean toward the patient
Visual cues, lip-reading
Eliminate distracting noises
Lower voice tone
Supplement with written material
Signing not too useful
Impaired vision
Well-lit room
Minimize glare
May have poor color vision
Dysarthria
Neurological
Dentures
Aphasia
Yes–no questions
Confusional state
Mental status exam
Patient may recognize problem/deny
See at different times to assess
Medications & medical conditions can
  cause confusion
Dementia is not part of normal aging
Touching (skin to skin)
Extremely useful even if unnecessary

Establish rapport/trust
Sit when speaking
Last name—permission otherwise
Explain what is to be accomplished
Utilize caring gestures
Eliminate physical barriers
Minimize distractions/interruptions
Culturally appropriate eye contact
Communicate concern/help

Reminiscence & life review
Not just "rambling"
Important in gaining trust
Provides insight into situation
Identifies things that give meaning

Underreporting of illness
May attribute symptoms to age

Aging is not a disease
CUPID (true physiological changes)
Cumulative, Universal, Progressive,
  Intrinsic, Deleterious
Ask specifically: weakness, weight loss,
  breathlessness, bowel/bladder
  function, hearing and visual losses,
  falls, memory loss, mood/depression

Multiplicity of illness
Rule rather than exception
Requires longer time, slower response
Requires patience (fatigue)
May need more than one visit
CC: multiple, overlapping, nonspecific
Organized record-keeping (POMR,
  problem list)

Altered presentation of illness
Symptoms may be nonspecific (different
  disease states)
Big Four: confusion, falls, immobility,
  incontinence
Fast heart, shortness of breath, physical
  disease as mental disorder
Symptoms change with aging
Reduced intensity of visceral pain
  (stoicism, mental impairment, pain
  appreciation)
Reduced sensation of breathlessness
Absence of thirst
Decreased fever response
Full-blown disease only clear as sudden,
  preterminal event

Disease itself may differ
Some "missing" diseases
Lethal diseases kill before old age
Reactions to infections less
Some viral diseases less; some more
Some diseases common in elderly
Cardiac (CAD, CHF, a fib)
Vascular (TIAs, CVAs, aneurysm,
  peripheral vascular disease)
Bone/joint (DJD, osteoporosis)
Skin
Urinary (BPH, atrophic vaginitis)
Gastrointestinal (colonic polyps &
  carcinomas, angiodysplasia,
  diverticular disease)
Neoplasms in general

Alternative history sources
Family, friends, neighbors
Other health professionals
Use other sources at later date
Degree of accuracy of source
Sensitivity when someone is present

Permission to have someone present
Address patient whenever possible
Attitude/knowledge of other sources
Separate interviews for privacy

Medication history
May be taking OTC drugs
Ability to afford and get medications
Ask patient to bring a list/containers
Include vitamins/herbal supplements
Check compliance
Child-resistant bottles difficult
Drug reactions/adverse interactions
Ask about and document allergies
Reactions may mimic stereotypes of "old
  age" (confusion, depression, anxiety,
  weakness, tremor, anorexia)
Is medication absolutely required?
If it makes patient feel better and does
  no harm, why not?

Nutritional history
High risk for malnutrition (widowed,
  homebound, acutely ill, mentally
  impaired, low income, NH)
Assess: access to food, fit of dentures,
  nutrient value, no. of meals
Taste (ageusia, dysgeusia)

Habits
Smoking & alcohol alter drug
  metabolism
Alcohol affects psychomotor & cognitive
  functions

Family history
Familial occurrence of illness
Witness disease and death of children

Psychosocial issues
Socialization/sig. relationships
Sexuality
Long-term care planning
Advance directives
Caregiving issues

Assessment of function
Sensory deficiencies
Physical: perform ADL, IADL
Support services (nursing, therapy)
Social: friends, relatives, church
Economics impacts on above
Nonverbal cues (personal hygiene)
"Describe a typical day for me."

Financial/economic issues
Concerns about costs of treatment
Resources for financial concerns

Fig. 3.1 Specific considerations in the history of the elderly patient. (Courtesy of University of Arizona College of Medicine.)

Reminiscence and life review
- Should not be viewed purely as "rambling."
- Leads to greater trust.
- Allows insight into patient reactions.
- Be sensitive to patient's needs.
- Find out what things give meaning to the patient's life.
- Allows insight into overall situation, which may influence final care.

Underreporting of illness
- "What can you expect at my age?" Older persons may attribute symptoms to age when they actually relate to treatable conditions.
- Combination of rationalization and denial.
- Never assume anything must be because of age.

True age-related physiological changes meet the CUPID criteria:
    C = Cumulative (the effects of the changes increase with successive additions).
    U = Universal (all humans show similar deficits with advancing age).
    P = Progressive (the changes take place gradually and are irreversible).
    I = Intrinsic (the changes must not be the result of a modifiable environment).
    D = Deleterious (the changes must reduce function).

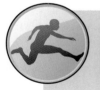

Aging is not a disease. Do not attribute to age symptoms that may be due to a treatable condition.

Ask specifically about:
- Weakness, weight loss, breathlessness.
- Bowel and bladder function (expect possible preoccupation with bowels).
- Hearing and visual losses.
- Falls.
- Memory loss, mood (depression).
- Specific questioning may bring out fears.

Multiplicity of illnesses
- Rule rather than exception.
- Requires longer time than with young patient.

- Illnesses, surgeries, injuries, medications (drug reactions, physicians, tests).
- Living situations.
- Losses.
- Family, friends (societal support).
- Job, income, home.
- Impaired physical skills that lead to decreased activity.
- Requires patience.
- Often have slower response times in answering questions.
- May fatigue more easily than younger persons.
- May necessitate two visits.
- CC may be multiple, overlapping, and nonspecific.
- 85% of ambulatory elderly have at least one chronic illness.
- Resist tendency to find a "unifying diagnosis"—multiple symptoms may really mean multiple illnesses.
- Any new complaint must be viewed superimposed on lengthy background.
- Look for change (may be subtle) in chronic complaint.

Multiplicity of illness is the rule rather than the exception in elderly patients. Resist the tendency to find a "unifying diagnosis." Multiple symptoms may really mean multiple illnesses.

Organized medical record-keeping is vital:
- Problem-oriented medical record (POMR).
- Particularly important is the problem list.

Altered presentation of illness
- Symptoms may be nonspecific due to many different disease states.
- Big four = confusion, falls, immobility, incontinence.
- Others: fast heart, shortness of breath.
- Physical disease (e.g., thyroid, COPD) may present as mental disorder.
- Some symptoms change with aging.
- Reduced intensity of visceral pain.

- Stoicism.
- Mental impairment.
- Physiology of pain appreciation.
- Reduced sensation of breathlessness.
- Absence of thirst.
- Decreased fever response.
- Full-blown disease may become clear only as sudden, preterminal event.

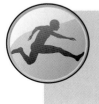

Symptoms in the elderly may be nonspecific due to many different disease states. The big four are confusion, falls, immobility, and incontinence.

Disease itself may differ:
- Some "missing" diseases, perhaps because some lethal diseases kill before old age (e.g., cystic fibrosis, Tay-Sachs disease).
- Reactions to infections decreased (e.g., erythema nodosum).
- Some viral diseases decrease (e.g., hepatitis); some increase (e.g., herpes zoster).

Particularly common diseases in the elderly
- Cardiac (coronary artery disease, congestive heart failure, atrial fibrillation).
- Vascular (transient ischemic attacks, cerebrovascular accidents, aneurysm, peripheral vascular disease).
- Bone and joint (degenerative joint disease, osteoporosis with or without fracture).
- Skin (actinic or seborrheic keratoses, basal cell epitheliomas).
- Genitourinary (benign prostatic hypertrophy, atrophic vaginitis).
- Gastrointestinal (colon polyps and carcinomas, angiodysplasia, diverticular disease, functional changes).
- Neoplasms in general.

Alternative history sources
- Include family, friends, and neighbors, other health professionals (useful also for extra attention, support, reinforcement), past medical records.

- May have to use these other sources at later time to gain an additional perspective.
- Define and recognize degree of accuracy of source.
- Be sensitive to interviewing patient with someone else present.
- Ask patient's permission to have caregiver or others present.
- Address questions to the patient whenever possible despite the presence of others.
- Note the attitude and knowledge of the other person regarding the patient.
- The end of the interview is a good time to dismiss the caregiver to allow the patient to discuss any private issues.
- Caregiver may be interviewed privately outside the room while the patient undresses.

Medication history
- May be taking over-the-counter drugs and prescriptions unknown to you.
- Ask patient to bring a list or containers of medications from home.
- Make sure vitamins and herbal supplements are included in inventory.
- Review medical records carefully.
- Assess ability to afford and get medication.
- Need to be sure of compliance; ask patients to bring in the bottles.
- Child-resistant containers can be difficult to open.
- Drug reactions and adverse interactions are 2–3 times more likely.
- Ask about medication allergies and document clearly.
- Reactions may mimic stereotypes of "old age" (e.g., forgetfulness, confusion, depression, anxiety, weakness, tremor, anorexia).
- Careful history of symptoms: Is any medication absolutely required?
- Be accepting of "minor addictions."
- Vitamin B_{12}, thyroid, other vitamin pills.
- If it makes patient feel better and does no harm, why not?

Nutritional history
- Factors that place elderly patients at high risk for malnutrition include homebound status, acute illness, recent widowhood, mental impairment, low income, and residence in nursing homes.
- Assess access to food (mobility, transportation), ability to prepare and eat (dentures), nutrient

value of diet, number of meals eaten, and taste (ageusia, dysgeusia).

Habits
- Smoking and alcohol may alter drug metabolism to a greater degree in elderly patients.
- Alcohol more profoundly affects psychomotor and cognitive functions in elderly people.

Family history
- Familial occurrence of illness.
- Impact on offspring.
- Senile dementia, coronary artery disease, diabetes mellitus, neoplasms, glaucoma.
- May catch something from the grandchildren.
- Often gets at health of significant other.
- Because of age, patients may have witnessed disease and death among their children.

Psychosocial issues
- Socialization activities/significant relationships.
- Sexuality.

- Long-term care planning.
- Advance directives.
- Caregiving issues.

Assessment of function
- Impact of sensory deficiencies.
- Physical stastus: ability to perform basic activities of daily living (ADLs) and instrumental activities of daily living (IADLs).
- Social status: friends, relatives, groups, home meals, church.
- Support services (e.g., nursing, physical or occupational therapy, home health).
- Economic status affects all of above.
- Look for nonverbal cues (e.g., tone of voice, personal hygiene).
- Ask the patient to "describe a typical day for me."

Financial/economic issues
- Elderly patients are often on "fixed incomes" and concerned about the fiscal aspects of treatment.
- Suggest resources that address financial concerns.

4. Presenting Problems: Cardiovascular System

Overview

In these next chapters we will look more closely at specific organ system-based interviews. We will use case studies to guide our work. Each of these chapters begins with an overview followed by specific patient cases. These clinical vignettes will help guide our work as we perform the medical interview. Some cases will provide details for each of the Sacred Seven questions, while others will present highlights from the patient's history.

As a central organ system responsible for delivering its cardiac output to the entire body, impaired cardiovascular system functioning can have significant and grave consequences. However, common symptoms of cardiovascular disease, such as chest pain, breathlessness, and fatigue, have noncardiac causes that are more common but less worrisome. It is the clinician's job, therefore, to triage among the various causes of these common symptoms. Moreover, due to the seriousness of the cardiac causes of these symptoms, patients often present with enormous anxieties.

The history taking is of critical importance as the physician searches for clues to rule in or rule out cardiovascular disease. Although many diagnostic and imaging tests are available, the clinician's history remains of prime importance. This history-taking skill enables the clinician to consider both the physiological and psychological causes of symptoms.

Cardiovascular system symptoms can result from obstructive disease (coronary artery thrombosis leading to the spectrum of angina through myocardial infarction), electrical disease (arrhythmia presenting as palpitations), mechanical disease (congestive heart failure due to left ventricular dysfunction presenting with shortness of breath), or autonomic disease (orthostatic hypotension presenting with fatigue). Finally, many psychological issues can present with somatic complaints such as chest pain.

Chest pain (cardiac)

History of present illness
Obtain a detailed account of the pain in a systematic manner, as described in Chapter 2, asking specifically about the features discussed below.

Location and radiation
Ask patients to indicate on themselves where exactly they experience the pain. Cardiac chest pain is typically retrosternal, but may only be present in the neck, throat, or arms (especially left arm). The pain may not radiate, but classically goes to the throat and left arm (see Fig. 4.1).

Quality
It is helpful to write down the exact words used by the patient. Cardiac chest pain is usually described as "tight," "crushing," "gripping," "like a band across my chest," "a dull ache." Patients often have difficulty finding words to describe abstract sensations such as pain, but it is important to try and ascertain its nature. You could give alternatives; for example, "Would you describe the pain as burning, stabbing, tightness, tearing sensation?" Remember to try and avoid leading the patient too much!

Often patients have had angina for a long time and may describe a pain as "like my angina, only worse," when experiencing a myocardial infarction.

 Your thumbnail sketch of the patient should include their risk factors for cardiovascular disease and, at best, what the patient's exercise tolerance is.

Make an attempt to distinguish the pain from other types of chest pain (Fig. 4.2). The main types of pain are:
- Cardiac.
- Pleuritic: sharp, stabbing, aggravated by coughing, deep breathing, or occasionally posture.

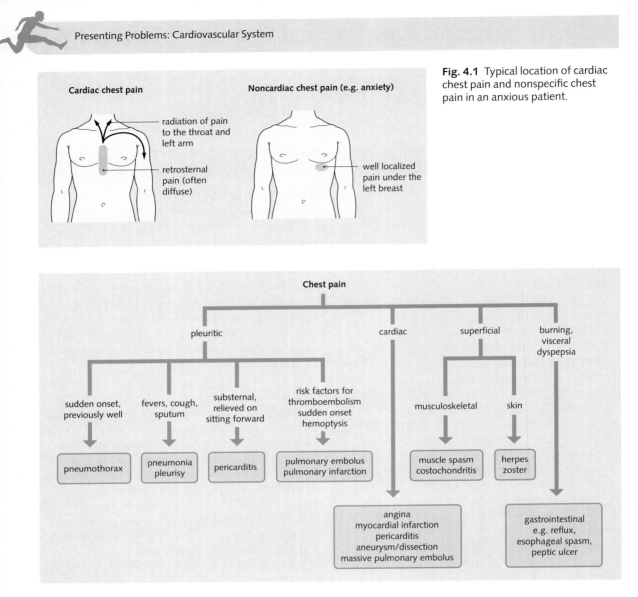

Fig. 4.1 Typical location of cardiac chest pain and nonspecific chest pain in an anxious patient.

Fig. 4.2 Differential diagnosis of chest pain.

- Gastrointestinal: often related to food ingestion, may be vague in character or described as burning, may be associated with an acid taste in the mouth.
- Musculoskeletal: usually easily recognized; the pain is often exaggerated by movement; there is often a good mechanical explanation, for example trauma or strain.
- Atypical diagnosis is partly by exclusion, partly by its atypical characteristics (e.g., sharp, lateral, and may be precipitated by stress or anxiety).

Severity

Ask the patient to compare the severity of the current pain to previous episodes of pain. A visual analog scale or a rating system of 1–10 may be helpful.

Setting or onset

Angina is typically provoked by exertion. If the pain is reproducible, try to find out the level of exertion necessary to induce it (e.g., walking up one flight of stairs, two or three blocks). Note if this level of exertion has changed recently. Ask specifically about other precipitating causes (e.g., stress, excitement, sexual intercourse, meals).

If this is the first episode of pain or its nature has changed, it is important to know what the patient was doing "immediately" before the onset of pain (e.g.,

Characteristics of angina and myocardial infarction		
Feature	Angina	Myocardial infarction
site	retrosternal, throat, left arm	retrosternal, throat, left arm
radiation	typically to the throat or left arm	typically to the throat or left arm
nature	"tight," "gripping," "a dull ache"	similar, but usually recognized as more severe
duration	short, usually a few minutes	usually greater than 30 minutes and only terminated by opiate analgesia
precipitation	exertion, stress, cold, emotion	usually none, but may have similar precipitants
relief	rest, NTG (rapid)	often none (opiates)
associated features	usually none	sweating, lightheadedness, palpitations, nausea, vomiting, sense of foreboding

Fig. 4.3 Characteristics of angina and myocardial infarction. NTG, nitroglycerin.

stable angina is provoked by a predictable stress, but unstable angina and myocardial infarction often occur at rest).

Timing
Angina usually lasts for only a few minutes and is typically relieved by rest. Patients often describe an urge to slow down or stop if they are walking at the onset of pain. Ask the patient exactly how long the pain takes to subside on rest—angina will usually resolve within seconds or at most a few minutes.

Modifying factors
If the patient takes nitroglycerin (NTG) tablets, inquire how quickly they seem to work. (Beware: some patients may have a false label of angina, and just because they are taking NTG tablets, it does not mean that the pain they are describing to you must be angina. Keeping an open mind is useful.) If the NTG does not help, make sure that the patient experiences some tingling under the tongue; otherwise, the NTG may have expired. A myocardial infarction usually causes pain lasting for longer than 20 minutes. It would be premature to ascribe such pain to stable angina without other good evidence.

Associated symptoms
Inquire specifically about any associated nausea, vomiting, sweating, shortness of breath, blackout, or collapse during the pain. If the patient describes palpitations, it is crucial to know whether they preceded the onset of pain as occasionally a

tachyarrhythmia may cause angina. Establish what the patient means by the term "palpitation" (ask them to tap out the rhythm). Make an attempt to distinguish between angina and myocardial infarction (Fig. 4.3).

Past medical history
Inquire specifically about the major caridac risk factors and previous episodes of angina or myocardial infarction. Record dates, events, and how the diagnosis was established (e.g., exercise test, hospital admission, angiography).

Cardiac risk factors
- Cigarette smoking. "Pack years" (i.e., the number of packs of cigarettes smoked daily multiplied by the years of smoking) is a useful concept. Current smokers have a significantly increased risk compared with ex-smokers.
- Hypertension.
- Diabetes mellitus.
- Hypercholesterolemia.
- Positive family history of ischemic heart disease.
- Other vascular disease (e.g., stroke, peripheral vascular disease).

The major risk factors interact, and the probability of disease is greatly increased if more than one is present.

Characteristics of common arrhythmias causing palpitations	
Rhythm	Typical features
ectopic beats	"I felt as though my heart missed a beat"; "a heavy thud"; usually due to awareness of post-extrasystolic beat
atrial fibrillation	"fast, irregular beating"; may be associated with dyspnea or chest pain, especially if fast rate
supraventricular tachycardia	rapid palpitation, often abrupt onset; may be associated with polyuria; may have rapid termination; patient may have learned to perform vagal maneuvers to terminate episode
ventricular tachycardia	often associated with shock, collapse, dyspnea, or progression to cardiac arrest; can be hard to distinguish from supraventricular arrhythmias as features overlap, and may even be asymptomatic; conversely, supraventricular tachycardia can cause shock, especially if rapid

Fig. 4.4 Characteristics of common arrhythmias causing palpitations.

Consider factors other than coronary artery disease that can cause angina (e.g., anemia, arrhythmia, previous valvular pathology, rheumatic fever).

Drug history

A full list of the medications the patient is currently taking is essential; however, it is important to also note the following:

- Have there been any recent changes?
- The effect of antianginal drugs on symptoms as well as side effects. In particular, does the pain resolve rapidly with sublingual NTG?
- Has concordance been good?
- Is the patient taking aspirin? Check that there are no contraindications (e.g., active ulceration, asthma provoked by aspirin).
- Consider the role of other drugs that might aggravate angina (e.g., theophylline, tricyclic antidepressants, wrong dose of thyroxine).

Social history

Inquire whether there have been any recent changes in lifestyle (e.g., financial difficulties, stress at home or work). These outside influences may be the precipitant for angina or a reason for developing a noncardiac chest pain. Ask how the chest pain has interfered with normal lifestyle.

Review of symptoms

A brief review of symptoms is important for various reasons:

- To exclude the gastrointestinal tract as the source of the symptoms (e.g., reflux esophagitis).
- Associated neurological symptoms may be provoked by decreased perfusion.

- To assess potential risks when considering invasive investigations or treatment (e.g., angiography or thrombolysis).
- To assess whether the patient has the mobility to tolerate an exercise tolerance test (ETT).
- To assess whether activity is limited by cardiac status or other factors such as poor mobility, obesity, or chronic lung disease.

Palpitations

Presenting complaint

Palpitation is an awareness of the heart beating. Different people mean different things when they say they have experienced palpitations.

History of present illness

It is essential to explore the event in great detail so that the underlying rhythm disturbance and functional consequences can be appreciated.

Nature of the palpitation

It is often possible to make a reasonable estimate of the underlying rhythm from the patient's description (Fig. 4.4)—for example, in response to questions such as "Can you describe what you experienced?," "Can you tap out the heart beat on the table?" The rate of the heart during the palpitation often provides a clue to the primary electrical disturbance (Fig. 4.5).

Duration and frequency of episodes

The functional impact on the patient may be revealed, as well as the likelihood of being able to

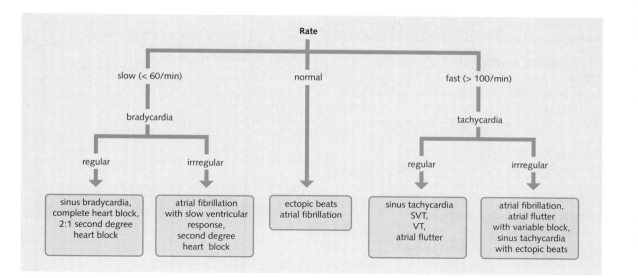

Fig. 4.5 Differential diagnosis of palpitations from the history. SVT, supraventricular tachycardia; VT, ventricular tachycardia.

"capture" the event on a 24-hour tape or event recorder.

Associated symptoms

Patients may have symptoms of cardiac decompensation, for example:

- Lightheadedness, fainting (syncope is due to poor cerebral perfusion and hypotension).
- Chest pain (angina).
- Sweating.

The presence of these symptoms should alert the physician and prompt more detailed investigation.

Events immediately preceding palpitation

It may be physiological to experience some palpitations after exertion or emotional stress, and this may be evident from the response to the question, "What were you doing immediately before the palpitations started?" If there was chest pain, find out whether the pain preceded the palpitation or coincided with its onset.

Past medical history

Review the possible underlying diseases that cause palpitations, including:

- Risk factors for ischemic heart disease.
- Thyroid disease (especially atrial fibrillation).
- Rheumatic fever.

Drug history

This is very important. Particular attention should be paid to drugs with proarrhythmic effects such as tricyclic antidepressants, digoxin, beta-blockers (and other antiarrhythmic agents), and theophylline. Review the response of the palpitations to therapy.

History of risk-taking behavior

Particular attention should be paid to alcohol consumption and caffeine-containing drinks. Use of recreational drugs (e.g., cannabis, ecstasy, amphetamines) may precipitate arrhythmias.

Summary of aims

The aims of the history for palpitations are as follows:

- To determine whether the rhythm is slow or fast, regular or irregular.
- To note any associated symptoms when the patient has the arrhythmia.
- To narrow the differential diagnosis of the arrhythmia. This is usually possible, but ultimately a diagnosis can only be made by an ECG recording at the time of symptoms.
- To assess whether the episodes are long enough and frequent enough and the patient is capable of using an event recorder or whether a 24-hour ECG is more appropriate if further investigation is needed.

Heart failure

Presenting complaint
Acute
Acute heart failure presents with severe shortness of breath, severe distress, production of copious pink, frothy sputum, and collapse.

Chronic
This presents with shortness of breath, limitation of exercise tolerance, ankle swelling, and fatigue.

History of present illness
The features of heart failure are usually distinctive enough to be recognized from the history alone, but airway obstruction can sometimes be confused with heart failure and may coexist with it. Lung disease often coexists with heart disease. The detailed history will clarify the presence of heart failure and establish its severity and possible etiology.

Chronicity of symptoms
Has the patient had a recent sudden decline suggestive of an ischemic event? Ask the patient, "What are you like normally?," "How many hospital admissions for this have you had in the past year?," and/or "Have you had to go to your primary care physician with worsening symptoms?"

Severity of symptoms
Attempt to quantify the patient's impairment so that a reproducible assessment can be made. Focus on tolerance to exercise and the limiting factor for exercise.

Exercise tolerance
It is often difficult to be precise, but patients should, with assistance, be able to give quantitative answers to questions such as "How many flights of stairs can you climb?," "How far can you walk on the flat and uphill?," or "Do you need help for any activities at home?" Try to quantify what factor limits exercise capacity (e.g., fatigue, coexisting lung disease, claudication). The severity of the heart failure may be graded according to the New York Heart Association classification (Fig. 4.6).

Limiting factors
Try to establish the limiting factor for exercise (e.g., dyspnea, fatigue, chest pain).

NHYA grading of severity of heart failure	
Grade	Severity of symptoms
I	unlimited exercise tolerance
II	symptomatic on extra exertion (e.g., stairs)
III	symptomatic on mild exertion (e.g., walking)
IV	symptomatic on minimal exertion or rest (e.g., washing)

Fig. 4.6 The New York Heart Association (NYHA) grading of severity of heart failure provides a simple but reproducible assessment with interobserver agreement.

Evidence of left heart failure
Inquire about features of pulmonary edema:
- Paroxysmal nocturnal dyspnea. This is a feature of acute pulmonary edema. Ask the patient, "Do you ever wake up in the night fighting for breath?" Patients often describe having to sit upright on the edge of the bed and/or throwing open the windows.
- Orthopnea. People may sleep with a few pillows for simple comfort or out of habit so it is important to find out if there has been any change. Ask the patient, "How many pillows do you need to sleep with and has this changed from usual?"

Evidence of right heart failure
Inquire about symptoms related to fluid overload, which may result in:
- Ascites.
- Peripheral edema (in severe cases male patients may have scrotal edema).
- Right upper quadrant discomfort (due to hepatic congestion).
- Nausea and poor appetite (due to bowel edema).

Past medical history
The most relevant features include:
- Risk factors for ischemic heart disease (see Chest pain, cardiac, p. 23 above).
- Previous cardiac investigations (e.g., echocardiography, angiography, exercise tolerance test).
- Other causes of left heart failure (e.g., rheumatic fever, valvular disease, cardiomyopathy), high output states (e.g., thyroid disease, Paget's disease, arteriovenous shunt, anemia).

- Other causes of right heart disease (e.g., chronic lung disease, pulmonary embolus).

Drug history

A full list of medication is needed, but focus on:

- Current therapy for heart failure, such as angiotensin-converting enzyme (ACE) inhibitors (cough may be a side effect or due to mild pulmonary edema), diuretics (assess concordance and find out whether there has been a recent change in dose).
- Negatively inotropic drugs (e.g., beta-blockers, verapamil, class I antiarrhythmic agents).
- Ask if the patient is on digoxin; if so, consider checking the level.

Social history

This section is very important. Assess daily activities, social support, mobility, etc. Review the patient's diet and appetite. Consider salt intake in edematous states. Does the patient have sufficient mobility to cope with an increased diuresis and avoid incontinence?

Deep vein thrombosis

Presenting complaint

Deep vein thrombosis (DVT) is a common condition. It is often asymptomatic; however, the most common features of presentation include:

- Calf pain.
- Leg swelling.
- Increased temperature of the leg.

Red tender leg

The history should be directed at finding risk factors for developing a DVT (an asterisk denotes the more important ones), which include:

- Pregnancy or puerperium.*
- Prolonged immobility (e.g. long-haul air travel).*
- Contraceptive pill.*
- Recent surgery.*
- Malignancy.
- Lower limb fractures.
- Heart failure.
- Dehydration.

Pulmonary embolism

Pulmonary embolus (PE) may be very difficult to diagnose, its presentation can vary from asymptomatic microemboli to sudden death caused by saddle embolism. The most common presentations are:

- Pleuritic chest pain.
- Shortness of breath.
- Hemoptysis.
- Collapse.

Thromboembolism is treatable and potentially fatal. It is underrecognized. A high index of suspicion is crucial.

Differential diagnosis of leg swelling or inflammation other than venous thrombosis	
Condition	Features
infection (cellulitis)	subacute onset; fever; lymphangitis may be present; ask about portal of entry for infecting organism
ruptured Baker's cyst	preceding arthritis or swelling of knee; acute onset
torn calf muscle	acute onset, often during exercise
congestive cardiac failure	dyspnea, fatigue, orthopnea; risk factors for ischemic heart disease; usually bilateral leg swelling
lymphatic obstruction	chronic; may be unilateral or bilateral
nephrotic syndrome	subacute or chronic leg swelling; bilateral; usually no features of inflammation

Fig. 4.7 Differential diagnosis of leg swelling or inflammation other than venous thrombosis.

History of present illness

If a PE is suspected, always ask specifically about risk factors suggestive of a DVT. In the presence of calf pain, investigate its features systematically (see Chapter 2). In particular, note any preceding symptoms, the speed of onset, any associated symptoms, and whether the pain is unilateral or bilateral. Figure 4.7 highlights some of the more discriminatory features in the history.

Almost 50% of DVTs do not produce local symptoms, so PE may be the presenting feature. Presentation may be nonspecific, and the differential diagnosis is wide. In the presence of pleuritic chest pain of undetermined etiology, do perform arterial blood gases and obtain a chest x-ray and an ECG.

5. Presenting Problems: Respiratory System

Overview

As with cardiovascular system disease, respiratory system disease presents with the common symptoms of cough, shortness of breath, and chest pain. Once again, the clinician's careful history often allows differentiation of the cause of the patient's symptoms.

Respiratory system disease can result from obstruction, infection, and mechanical causes. Airway obstruction or bronchoconstriction in asthma can lead to shortness of breath. The obstructive character of a pulmonary embolus or a malignant lesion also causes shortness of breath. Viral, bacterial, parasitic, or fungal organisms can cause the cough of pneumonia. These different etiologies demonstrate varying degrees of fever, productive cough, and character of the sputum. The alveolar destruction in chronic obstructive pulmonary disease (COPD) causes the patient to be short of breath and results in a specific breathing pattern. Finally, the fluid in a pleural effusion can impair gas exchange and at times diaphragmatic excursion, also leading to shortness of breath.

Asthma

Presenting complaint

Can you actually obtain a history from the patient? If the patient cannot talk in sentences, you have identified a medical emergency and you must seek help. However, the most common presentations include episodic wheeze, shortness of breath, or a (nocturnal) cough.

History of present illness

If the patient presents with an acute attack, investigate this attack in detail. Obtain a systematic, chronological account of the recent deterioration, focusing on:
- Severity: try to quantify in simple terms (e.g., unable to perform vigorous exercise, difficulty climbing stairs, unable to speak a complete sentence, being kept awake at night).

 An acute asthma attack is often frightening for both the patient and the attending physician. The patient is often too dyspneic to provide much history. The priority is to make a rapid assessment and institute effective therapy. A more detailed history can be obtained once the patient is stable.

- Symptoms (e.g., wheeze, cough, dyspnea).
- Time course (hours or days).
- Onset and precipitating events (e.g., exercise, emotional stress, viral illness, house dust, pets).
- Intervention during present attack and response (e.g., nebulized bronchodilators, steroids).
- Reason for seeking medical attention at this stage.

Often asthma control has deteriorated chronically and insidiously. Ask the following questions:
- "Is there anything that you could do 6 months ago that you couldn't manage before this attack?"
- "Have you reduced your exercise over the past few months?"
- Has the patient been seeing his/her primary care physician about the asthma?

Past medical history
Baseline asthma control
It is helpful to gain an awareness of the background control. In addition to allowing an assessment of disease severity, it may reveal information about the patient's understanding of the disease. Ask about:
- Usual exercise tolerance. Try to quantify as described above. (Young patients should have unlimited exercise capacity. Older patients often have coexisting morbidity.)
- Frequency of attacks.
- Best recorded peak expiratory flow rate (PEFR). Ideally all asthma patients should have their own peak flow meter and know their baseline PEFR.

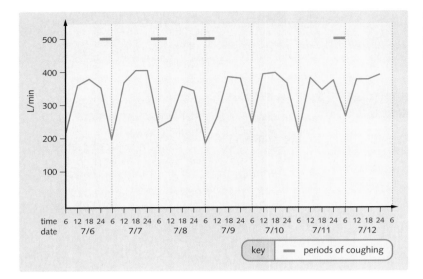

Fig. 5.1 An example of a peak flow recording from an adolescent with poor asthma control. Note the presence of cough at night and "morning dips."

- Usual precipitating factors (e.g., pollen, stress, exercise, dust, pollution).
- Usual medication (see below).
- Usual response to therapy during exacerbations. For example, ask "Is this the worst attack you've ever had?," "Would you normally expect your asthma attacks to get better after using a nebulizer?"
- Previous hospital admissions. For example, ask "Have you ever been admitted to hospital with asthma?," "Have you ever needed to be put on a ventilator?"
- Symptoms suggestive of poor baseline control. This is very important and underrecognized (e.g., "morning dips," poor sleep, nocturnal cough, time off work or school). An example of a peak flow chart from a child with poor control is illustrated in Fig. 5.1.

Other atopic conditions

Ask about other atopic conditions such as eczema, hay fever, urticaria.

Coexisting respiratory disease

Coexisting respiratory disease is particularly important in patients who present later in life, as it may be hard to distinguish asthma from chronic obstructive pulmonary disease (COPD) on the basis of the history.

Drug history

Obtain a full list of medication. Ask specifically:
- Does the patient have a nebulizer at home?
- Does the patient use bronchodilators?
- Does the patient take steroids, inhaled or oral?

Ask patients to demonstrate their inhaler technique. It is possible to quantify inhaler techniques as in Fig. 5.2. Find out whether pulmonary function tests have been performed to assess airway reversibility, and responses to different agents, especially for older patients for whom it may be difficult to define the relative components of asthma and COPD to the overall morbidity. Consider medication that may aggravate the symptoms (e.g., beta-blockers, aspirin).

Inhaler technique scoring	
Prepares device (e.g., shakes inhaler)	1
Exhales fully	1
Activates and inhales	1
Holds breath for several seconds	1

Fig. 5.2 Inhaler technique scoring (total out of 4).

Social history

Review how the asthma is interfering with lifestyle for both older and young patients (e.g., school activities, absenteeism from work, limitation in sports, difficulty walking to the shops).

History of risk-taking behavior

Always specifically inquire about smoking. During an exacerbation, it is timely to offer sensitive advice about smoking! Ask whether anyone in the patient's household is a smoker.

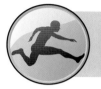

No one with asthma should smoke!

Review of systems

Focus on other diseases that may limit exercise tolerance, especially cardiovascular, respiratory pathology, and arthritis.

Remember that asthma is a potentially fatal disease. The morbidity and mortality rates are high but can be overcome by better supervision, objective assessment, better patient understanding and participation in his or her management, and appropriate use of steroids.

Chronic obstructive pulmonary disease

History of present illness

Obtain a detailed history of chest symptoms. In an acute exacerbation, patients usually present following a cold with a deterioration of dyspnea in association with a productive cough and discolored sputum. Outline a detailed history of the present attack following the usual systematic approach to explore:

- Time course.
- Treatment given and effects.
- Functional impact on lifestyle.

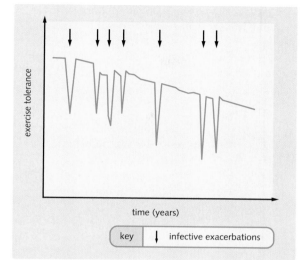

Fig. 5.3 Exercise tolerance in a patient with COPD.

- Any hospital admissions in the last year for COPD.
- Has the patient been seeing his/her primary care physician with the problem.

Obtain a thorough history of baseline function, trying to be as objective as possible. For example, ask:
- "How far can you walk?"
- "Can you climb one flight of stairs easily?"
- "Do you get short of breath dressing?"

It is typical for a patient with COPD to have a pattern of chronically deteriorating exercise tolerance punctuated with acute declines during an infective exacerbation (Fig. 5.3). These may be seasonal, with an increased frequency in the winter months.

Sputum production and cough are characteristic. Try to quantify the usual amount per day and its characteristics (e.g., a teaspoonful, a cupful).

Chronic bronchitis is defined on the basis of the history of cough productive of sputum on most days for 3 consecutive months for at least 2 years. Emphysema is a pathological diagnosis of dilatation and destruction of the lungs distal to the terminal bronchioles. In practice, these conditions coexist.

Consider the possibility of cor pulmonale in a patient with severe disease who describes ankle swelling.

Ascertain aggravating factors (e.g., cold weather, pollution, exertion).

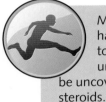 Many patients with COPD have a reversible component to their disease. This is underrecognized but can be uncovered by a formal trial of steroids.

Find out whether a satisfactory attempt has been made to establish the diagnosis:
- Have lung function tests been performed to assess airway reversibility?
- Have arterial blood gases been performed when the patient is well?

 Blood gases for assessment of COPD should be taken 3 months after any acute illness.

Past medical history

These patients may have multiple medical problems, which should be recorded, but specifically ask about:
- Previous hospital admissions with acute exacerbations of COPD. Record the frequency, especially within the last year.
- Other smoking-related diseases (e.g., ischemic heart disease, peripheral vascular disease, strokes, hypertension).
- Other causes of lung disease (e.g., occupational exposure to dusts, bronchiectasis due to previous tuberculosis, childhood whooping cough).
- Asthma. There may be a reversible component to the disease.

Drug history

Review medication prescribed for COPD:
- Bronchodilators (inhalers and nebulizers).

- Home oxygen. Who initiated therapy and on what evidence? How many hours a day is it being used? Oxygen therapy should be used for 16 hours per day to prevent cor pulmonale. It is not for improving oxygen saturations per se.
- Steroids. Does the patient have a record of use?
- Review inhaler technique.

Social history

This is particularly important for these patients as they often have significant limitation of exercise tolerance and rely heavily upon support from family, friends, and state. Ask, for example, whether the patient is receiving any benefits. Consider all aspects of daily living.

History of risk-taking behavior

Obtain a detailed smoking history as this is undoubtedly a smoking-related disease in the vast majority of patients. Remember that the patient must not smoke if they are using home oxygen!

A detailed occupational history may be important if there is any doubt about the patient's ability to continue working or the etiology of the lung disease. For example:
- Exposure to inorganic dusts (coalminer's lung, silicosis, asbestosis).
- Occupational asthma (isocyanates, rosin fumes).
- Extrinsic allergic bronchiolar alveolitis (farmworkers, hypersensitivity pneumonitis).

Review of systems

Many patients with COPD have multiple pathologies related to their smoking, so a thorough review of their symptoms may raise suspicions of previously unrecognized conditions (e.g., ischemic heart disease, malignancy, renal disease, peripheral vascular disease).

 Meticulous and realistic assessment of baseline function is essential. Without this, it is impossible to make difficult decisions about appropriate treatment and to set realistic goals of therapy.

Clues to the underlying cause of pneumonia	
Organism	**Features from history**
*Streptococcus pneumoniae**	most frequent identifiable infecting organism in community-acquired pneumonia; associated with herpes labialis, commonly prominent fever and pleuritic pain; often abrupt onset in previously fit individual
*Mycoplasma pneumoniae**	occurs in epidemics with a 3–4-year periodicity; usually occurs in previously fit people, often young adults; may be preceded by a prodromal illness with headache and malaise; may be prominent extrapulmonary features (e.g., nausea, vomiting, myalgia, rash)
*Hemophilus influenzae**	most common bacterial pneumonia following influenza; associated with underlying lung disease (especially COPD)
Legionella pneumophila	associated with institutional outbreaks (e.g., hospitals, hotels); may be associated with mental confusion or gastrointestinal symptoms; typically causes a dry cough
Coxiella burnetii	contact with farm animals
Chlamydia psittaci	contact with infected birds ("Do you have a sick parrot?")
Staphylococcus aureus	associated with preceding influenza, intravenous drug abusers, patient is often very ill
Gram-negative organisms	hospitalized patients; may be community-acquired in elderly or diabetics; *Branhamella catarrhalis* is associated with exacerbations of COPD
Pneumocystis carinii, cytomegalovirus, Nocardia asteroides, Mycobacterium avium intracellulare	acquired immunodeficiency syndrome (AIDS); transplant recipients; chemotherapy
Mycobacterium tuberculosis	weight loss, chronic cough, foreign travel, infected family member

Fig. 5.4 Clues to the underlying cause of pneumonia. Asterisks denote the more common organisms.

Chest infection

History of present illness

Perform a detailed inquiry about presenting symptoms, adopting a methodical approach. Ask specifically about symptoms referable to the respiratory tract as follows:

- Cough: duration, whether productive or dry.
- Sputum production: quantity, color, recent changes if the patient has a productive cough.
- Dyspnea: obtain a quantitative account of exercise tolerance at baseline and during the current illness.
- Wheeze.
- Pleuritic chest pain: a common feature of pneumonia, but be aware of the possibility of a pulmonary embolus.
- Fever.

If symptoms are prolonged, recurrent, or associated with weight loss, consider the possibility of an underlying malignancy, especially in a smoker.

Ask about associated symptoms that have immediately preceded or coincided with the illness (especially gastrointestinal). These may give additional clues to the infecting organism causing pneumonia. Figure 5.4 illustrates how a detailed history may help to identify the microbiological cause of a pneumonic illness.

Drug history

Ask specifically about antibiotics used to treat this and any recent episode and the duration of use as the response to therapy may give a clue to the infecting agent as well as the likelihood of obtaining a positive blood culture. For example:

- Resistance of *Mycoplasma* to penicillin.
- Resistance of tuberculosis or *Pneumocystis* to repeated courses of antibiotics.

Find out if the patient is taking immuno-suppressive medication (e.g., those taking steroids, transplant recipients) (Fig. 5.4).

Social history

Relevant clues may be provided by a travel history and details of hobbies (e.g., involving pets) and occupation. Clearly it is important to assess the functional impact of the disease on patients and their families so that appropriate therapeutic and management decisions can be made.

History of risk-taking behavior

- Risk factors for HIV infection.
- Smokers are more likely to decompensate earlier in the course of the illness.

6. Presenting Problems: Abdominal

Overview

Once again, common symptoms define diseases of the abdominal system. These common symptoms include abdominal pain, gastrointestinal bleeding, infections, and disorders of peristalsis, including diarrhea and constipation. Other common symptoms related to the abdominal system include difficulty swallowing, nausea, vomiting, anorexia, and weight loss. The astute clinician is called on again to differentiate organic from functional disease.

Acute abdominal pain

History of present illness

A very careful history needs to be elicited as it will form the foundation for a working hypothesis and differential diagnosis and rational subsequent investigation.

On the basis of the history, abdominal pain can be divided into three types:

- Visceral.
- Somatic.
- Referred.

Visceral (deep) pain

This is dull, poorly localized pain referred to the midline. The site of pain is derived from its embryological origin (foregut, midgut, hindgut) (Fig. 6.1).

Somatic (peritoneal) pain

This is sharp, severe, and more precisely localized pain. It occurs when the disease process involves the surrounding peritoneum and mesentery.

Referred pain

This is the perception of sensory stimuli at a distance from its source (e.g., acute cholecystitis causing diaphragmatic irritation with the patient feeling pain over the right shoulder). The characteristics of the pain should be reviewed in a systematic manner as for other forms of pain (e.g., see "Chest pain"). There are several key areas which should always be investigated. How to take a pain history is outlined in Chapter 2.

Location and radiation

Define the initial location of the pain and whether it has subsequently moved (e.g., acute appendicitis). This is of great importance as certain disease processes tend to cause pain localized to a defined region of the abdomen (Fig. 6.2). Flank pain, for example, radiates to the groin in renal colic.

Timing

Sudden-onset pain suggests a vascular event (e.g., rupture of an abdominal aortic aneurysm), or perforation of a viscus: "One moment I was feeling fine, the next I was doubled up with pain!"

Quality

The pain may change character, indicating progression of the pathology (e.g., transition of colicky pain to constant pain suggests transition of visceral to peritoneal involvement in acute appendicitis).

Severity

Is the pain getting worse, better, or staying at the same intensity? "If 0 equals no pain, and 10 is the worst pain you have ever experienced, what value would you give this pain?"

Setting or onset

Colicky pain occurs when there is a pathological process in a smooth muscular tube (e.g., small and large bowel, ureter, fallopian tube). Ask whether the patient has had previous similar episodes.

Modifying factors

It is often apparent from first seeing patients what type of pain they have (e.g., patients with peritonitis lie still, patients with renal colic are often very restless). Certain foods may aggravate pain (e.g., fatty foods aggravate abdominal pain due to gallstones). The pain of pancreatitis is characteristically relieved by sitting forward, duodenal ulcer pain may be relieved by eating, and antacids or sleeping upright may relieve the pain of reflux esophagitis.

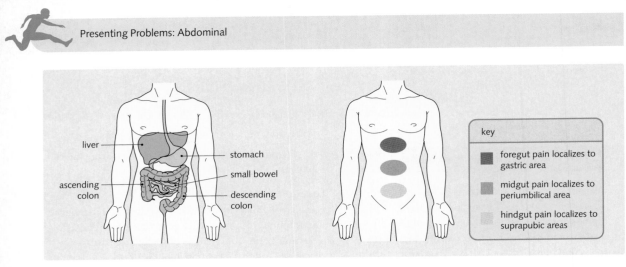

Fig. 6.1 The site of abdominal pain is related to the embryological development of the foregut, midgut, and hindgut.

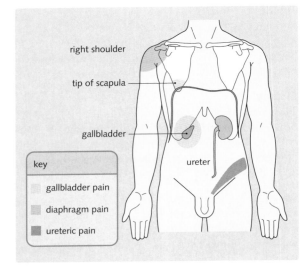

Fig. 6.2 Typical sites of radiation pain for pain originating in the gallbladder, diaphragm, and ureter.

Other symptoms

Review other symptoms referable to the abdominal system:

- When was the patient's last bowel movement, and when was flatus last passed? This is particularly relevant if partial or complete obstruction is suspected.
- Change in bowel habit. This is likely to reflect a large bowel pathology (e.g., carcinoma, inflammatory bowel disease).
- Vomiting. Establish the nature of the vomitus (e.g., blood, bile, "coffee grounds," feculent) and when it occurs in relation to eating.
- "Do you still feel hungry?" This question is useful for discriminating nonserious pathology as the majority of patients with serious intra-abdominal disease have anorexia.
- Abdominal distension.
- Appetite and weight loss. Chronic weight loss is suggestive of an underlying malignancy. It is useful to ask if the patient's clothes still fit.
- Dysphagia. Ask the patient to point to where the food appears to stick. Establish whether the dysphagia is for food alone or food and drink. Inquire whether there is associated pain on swallowing.
- Are any foods particularly associated with pain (e.g., fatty foods)?
- Regurgitation, flatulence, heartburn, dyspepsia. Ask about these symptoms if peptic ulcer disease, gastroesophageal reflux, or gallstone disease is suspected.
- Urinary symptoms. Frequency and dysuria may suggest a urinary tract infection. Nocturia, urgency, and hesitancy are consistent with prostatic enlargement.
- History of trauma. Have a low index of suspicion for a splenic or hepatic tear.

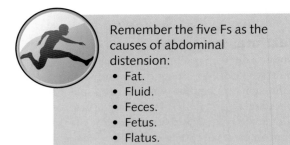

Remember the five Fs as the causes of abdominal distension:
- Fat.
- Fluid.
- Feces.
- Fetus.
- Flatus.

Fig. 6.3 Medical conditions that can mimic a "surgical abdomen." The history may distinguish medical conditions masquerading as surgical problems. Asterisks indicate the more common conditions.

Medical conditions that can mimic a "surgical abdomen"	
Medical condition presenting as abdominal pain	**Features**
myocardial infarction (MI)*	especially inferior MI; may have paradoxical bradycardia; risk factors for ischemic heart disease
angina*	usually epigastric
chest infection*	especially lower lobe pneumonia; previous respiratory symptoms; pleurisy
diabetic ketoacidosis*	especially young patients; decreased level of consciousness; preceding polyuria, poldipsia, weight loss; positive family history
acute pyelonephritis*	dysuria, hematuria, frequency; flank pain versus central abdominal pain; history of renal stones
hypercalcemia	often elderly; "bones, stones, moans, and groans"
sickle cell crisis	ethnic origin, usually known history

Chapter 16 deals with how to take a gynecological history from a woman if a gynecological cause is suspected.

Consider the possibility of pregnancy in all women of childbearing age.

It is particularly important to include a cardiovascular and respiratory history as several medical conditions can cause acute abdominal pain (Fig. 6.3).

Past medical history
Obtain a detailed history, paying particular attention to:
- Previous operations (e.g., adhesions, recurrent pathology).
- Recent myocardial infarction or cardiac arrhythmias: mesenteric embolus, especially in association with atrial fibrillation.

- Psychiatric history: patients will not volunteer this information. A high index of suspicion together with old notes is needed for a diagnosis.
- Hypothyroidism.
- Constipation.

Drug history
Obtain a full list of medications. Pay attention to nonsteroidal anti-inflammatory drugs (NSAIDs) and steroids. Also consider drugs that may provoke constipation (e.g., opiates, tricyclic antidepressants, antimuscarinic agents, antiparkinsonism therapy).

Family history
There may be a positive family history of inflammatory bowel disease or bowel carcinoma.

Social history
For diarrheal illnesses, consider foreign travel (e.g., amebiasis, typhoid, giardiasis) or food poisoning (ask "Are any of your friends or family also affected?"). The patient often has a strong inkling that symptoms have been caused by food and may be able to pinpoint exactly the suspect meal.

History of risk-taking behavior
Alcohol history is extremely important (e.g., for peptic ulcer, pancreatitis).

If the patient may need an operation, do not forget to ask when he or she last had food or drink. In all cases it is mandatory to give analgesia at the earliest opportunity. It does not make interpretation of physical signs difficult, and patients give better histories if they are less distracted.

Acute diarrheal illness

History of present illness

Diarrhea is a symptom and not a disease. Therefore, it is important to establish the underlying cause. Ask about the nature of the stools, frequency, and events surrounding the episode. Important features to ask about include:

- Recent ingestion of undercooked meat, shellfish, unpasteurized milk, stream water (i.e., food poisoning).
- Associated abdominal pain and vomiting. Is the patient likely to need intravenous fluids?
- Is the pain relieved by defecation?
- Is there blood, pus, or mucus in the stool?
- Are the stools pale and frothy? (i.e. steatorrhea).
- Duration of symptoms (e.g., hours, weeks, days). Different illnesses may present acutely or subacutely.
- Weight loss or anorexia.
- Recent return from a foreign country (e.g., amebiasis, giardiasis).
- Allergy to gluten products.
- Symptoms of thyrotoxicosis (e.g., heat intolerance, agitation, palpitations); thyrotoxicosis occasionally presents with diarrhea.

Past medical history

Obtain a detailed history, paying particular attention to:

- Previous operations (e.g., short bowel syndrome, gastrectomy and vagotomy dumping).
- Inflammatory bowel disease.

Drug history

The drug history is particularly important as drugs commonly contribute to a diarrheal state. Common culprits include antibiotics, laxative abuse (may be surreptitious), and magnesium-containing antacids.

Family history

Inquire about inflammatory bowel disease, carcinoma of the bowel, and celiac disease.

Social history

An infective etiology is suggested if friends or relatives have a similar illness. If the patient is dehydrated, frail, or responsible for childcare, consider whether admission is indicated.

The more common causes of diarrhea are listed in Fig. 6.4.

Jaundice

Presenting complaint

Jaundice presents with yellow discoloration, which is initially often not noticed by the patient.

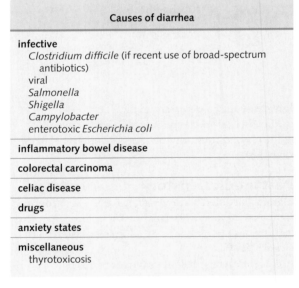 Painless jaundice in a patient over 55 should be considered to be a cancer of the head of the pancreas until proved otherwise. In patients under 55 it is most likely to be hepatitis A.

Causes of diarrhea
infective
Clostridium difficile (if recent use of broad-spectrum antibiotics)
viral
Salmonella
Shigella
Campylobacter
enterotoxic *Escherichia coli*
inflammatory bowel disease
colorectal carcinoma
celiac disease
drugs
anxiety states
miscellaneous
thyrotoxicosis

Fig. 6.4 Causes of diarrhea.

History of present illness

The history of a jaundiced patient is very challenging as the pathophysiology is so varied. It is helpful to review the pathophysiology of jaundice (Figs. 6.5 and 6.6). Focus on the major features.

Onset

Who noticed the jaundice (e.g., patient, family, abnormal blood test)? Establish the time course (e.g., acute onset in fulminant hepatitis A, insidious progression in biliary stricture).

Associated symptoms

It is often possible to narrow down the differential diagnosis of jaundice by a detailed history. Many causes of jaundice have typical features. The usual classification is prehepatic, hepatocellular, or posthepatic. Often the features of hepatocellular and obstructive jaundice overlap.

Prehepatic jaundice (hemolytic)

Jaundice is usually a minor component. The illness is often dominated by symptoms of anemia (e.g., fatigue, dyspnea, angina, and palpitations [in older patients]). It may be associated with gallstones (pigment stones). On specific questioning patients report normal-colored stool and urine. Patients may be transfusion-dependent. Consider the possible causes (i.e., abnormal red cells or immune-mediated hemolysis).

Examples of abnormal red cells occur in:

- Congenital spherocytosis (northern Europe).
- Glucose-6-phosphate dehydrogenase (G6PD) deficiency (West Africa, Mediterranean, Middle East, Southeast Asia).
- Sickle cell anemia (sub-Saharan Africa).
- Thalassemia (Mediterranean, Middle East, India, Southeast Asia).

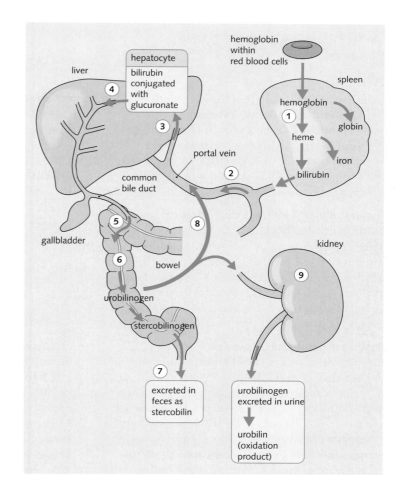

Fig. 6.5 The production, circulation, and clearance of bilirubin (see also Fig. 6.6).

Production and clearance of bilirubin		
Stage	Description	Example of pathology
1	hemoglobin within the red cells broken down within the spleen producing non-water-soluble unconjugated bilirubin	excessive breakdown (e.g., hemolytic anemia)
2	unconjugated bilirubin transported in the blood to the liver	
3	uptake of bilirubin by the hepatocytes and transfer to the smooth endoplasmic reticulum	drug toxicity; Gilbert's syndrome; Rotor's syndrome
4	conjugation with glucuronate	Crigler–Najjar syndrome
5	excretion of conjugated bilirubin in the bile into the small bowel	biliary obstruction (defect may occur at level of hepatocyte, bile canaliculi, or bile duct)
6	breakdown within bowel to stercobilinogen (urobilinogen)	
7	oxidation of stercobilinogen to stercobilin (causes brown coloration of feces) and excretion	white stool in cholestatic jaundice
8	absorption of urobilinogen; most goes through enterohepatic recirculation	
9	small amount of urobilinogen (water-soluble) reaches systemic circulation and excreted via the kidney	large amounts of urinary urobilinogen detectable if severe hemolysis or liver damage saturates the liver's capacity for enterohepatic recirculation

Fig. 6.6 Production and clearance of bilirubin.

Causes of immune-mediated hemolysis include:
- Drugs (e.g., methyldopa, penicillin).
- Incompatible blood transfusion (acute onset).
- Warm autoantibodies (e.g., systemic lupus erythematosus, lymphoproliferative disorders).
- Cold agglutinins (e.g., infectious mononucleosis, *Mycoplasma*).

Hepatocellular jaundice (inability to excrete bilirubin into the bile)

This is often dominated by symptoms of liver dysfunction (e.g., malaise, anorexia, right upper quadrant discomfort, abdominal distension, loss of libido, confusion). The list of diseases that may be responsible is vast, but the more important causes are illustrated in Fig. 6.7.

Posthepatic jaundice (cholestatic)

The patient may complain of pruritus due to the deposition of bile salts. It is usually, but not always, relentlessly progressive rather than episodic. There is often a history of pale stools and dark urine due to a lack of stercobilinogen in the stool and retention of conjugated bilirubin. It is important to recognize extrahepatic causes of obstructive jaundice as these are often amenable to surgical intervention (Fig. 6.8).

Past medical history

Obtain a detailed history, paying particular attention to more recent events:
- Alcohol abuse: recent binge.
- Ulcerative colitis: may suggest the presence of sclerosing cholangitis.
- Recent viral illness: Gilbert's syndrome, hepatitis A or B.
- Gallstones: either a cause of jaundice or a consequence of chronic hemolysis.

Drug history

An extremely careful drug history should be taken as drugs may have precipitated the jaundice. In addition, certain drugs need to be avoided or used with care in liver disease. For example:
- Drugs causing hemolysis by acting as haptens (e.g., penicillin, sulfonamides), direct autoimmune effect (e.g., methyldopa), precipitating hemolysis in G6PD deficiency (e.g., primaquine, nitrofurantoin).
- Drugs causing hepatocellular damage (e.g., paracetamol overdose, alcohol, isoniazid).
- Drugs causing intrahepatic cholestasis (e.g., estrogens, phenothiazines).

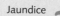

Causes of hepatocellular jaundice

Cause	Examples
viral*	hepatitis A* (common, especially in endemic areas may occur in epidemics; may present acutely); hepatitis B* (common in endemic areas, e.g., Southeast Asia; ask specifically about risk factors for bloodborne infections); hepatitis C* (becoming more common; ask about blood transfusions, shared needles in drug addicts; usually chronic insidious illness)
alcoholic*	common; often presents as acute hepatitic illness
drugs*	common in hospitalized patients (e.g., rifampicin, isoniazid, prolonged course of antibiotics, paracetamol overdose, etc.)
cirrhosis*	of any etiology (e.g., alcohol, biliary, hemochromatosis, etc.)
malignant infiltration*	primary or secondary (especially bronchus, bowel, breast)
congenital	for example Gilbert's syndrome* (common and mild); Crigler–Najjar syndrome
acute fatty liver of pregnancy	rare
inherited disorders	for example α-1-antitrypsin deficiency, Wilson's disease, etc.

Fig. 6.7 Causes of hepatocellular jaundice. Asterisks indicate the more common causes.

Causes of posthepatic jaundice

Cause	Features from the history
gallstones*	common; often intermittent history of biliary colic or rigors; "fat, female, forty, fertile"
carcinoma of head of pancreas*	weight loss; pain; relentless progression
pancreatitis*	acute onset; patient often very ill
benign stricture of common bile duct	may mimic carcinoma of the pancreas
sclerosing cholangitis	associated ulcerative colitis
cholangiocarcinoma	

Fig. 6.8 Causes of posthepatic jaundice. Asterisks indicate the more common causes.

- Drugs causing gallstones (e.g., oral contraceptives, clofibrate).

Social history

Reviewing the patient's lifestyle may provide many clues to the etiology. A travel history is particularly pertinent (e.g., to an area where hepatitis A is endemic). Social contacts with hepatitis A may be apparent if there has been an epidemic. Finally, review the patient's occupation and hobbies (e.g., leptospirosis in sewage workers or farmers, exposure to toxins by workers with organic solvents, hepatitis B in healthcare workers on dialysis units).

History of risk-taking behavior

A detailed alcohol history is essential for acute alcoholic hepatitis and cirrhosis. Risk factors for bloodborne infections (e.g., intravenous drug abuse, unprotected persistent sexual intercourse, multiple blood transfusions) should be considered (e.g., for hepatitis B or C, or HIV infection). Cigarette smoking may point to malignant disease.

Family history

A family history is particularly relevant for younger patients (e.g., for Gilbert's syndrome, hemoglobinopathies, Wilson's disease).

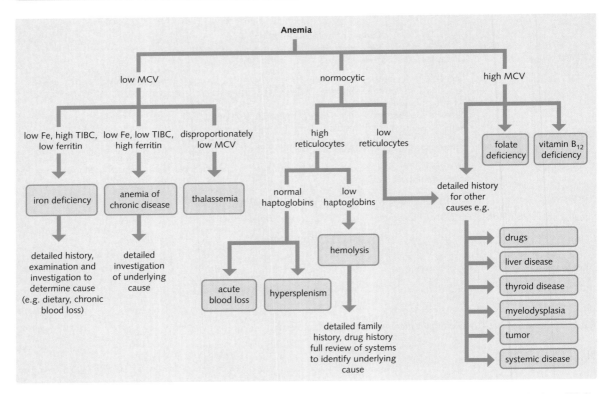

Fig. 6.9 Algorithm for the differential diagnosis of anemia based on the mean corpuscular volume (MCV). Fe, iron; TIBC, total iron-binding capacity.

Review of systems

The differential diagnosis is broad, so a complete systems inquiry is needed.

> The differential diagnosis of jaundice is broad. A detailed history is needed to focus further investigations.

Anemia

Presenting complaint

May be insidious (with lethargy, pallor, tired all the time) or an incidental finding on blood test.

History of present illness

Review symptoms related to anemia. Ask specifically about:
- Lethargy.
- Exercise tolerance.

- Palpitations.
- Angina and intermittent claudication (older patients).
- Dyspnea.

Try to establish the duration of symptoms; the causes of acute and chronic anemia are different. For example, ask "When did you last feel completely well?" Obtain the results of previous laboratory investigations; they may help in differentiating acute and chronic causes (Fig. 6.9).

Usually the result of the blood smear will be available. It is helpful to categorize anemia according to the mean corpuscular volume (MCV) (Fig. 6.10) as:
- Hypochromic microcytic.
- Normochromic normocytic.
- Macrocytic.

Past medical history

Take an extensive history. Ask specifically about the following conditions, including symptoms relating to:

Causes of anemia	
Causes	**Features**

hypochromic
  iron deficiency*
 	
  thalassemia trait and disease
  anemia of chronic disease*
  congenital sideroblastic anemia
	overwhelmingly the most common cause of anemia, usually a chronic insidious pattern (e.g., dietary, chronic blood loss)
	disproportionately low MCV; Mediterranean; family history
	may have normal MCV
	rare

normochromic normocytic
  hemolytic anemia*
  aplastic anemia
  anemia of chronic disease
	often variable red cell indices
	may have variable MCV due to reticulocytosis (e.g., G6PD deficiency, drug-induced, etc.)
	usually multifactorial causes (e.g., malignancy, chronic renal failure, connective tissue disease, etc.)

macrocytic
  vitamin B_{12} deficiency*
  folate deficiency*
  alcohol*
  hypothyroidism
  liver disease
  reticulocytosis
  myelodysplasia
  acquired sideroblastic anemia
	common, megaloblastic (e.g., pernicious anemia, veganism)
	common, megaloblastic (e.g., nutritional, malabsorption, pregnancy)
	the most common cause of an elevated MCV
	
	rare
	rare

Fig. 6.10 Causes of anemia. Asterisks indicate the more common causes. G6PD, glucose-6-phosphate dehydrogenase.

- Peptic ulceration or indigestion: blood loss causing iron deficiency.
- Malignancy: chronic disease, marrow infiltration, blood loss.
- Renal disease: chronic disease, blood loss, hemolysis, erythropoietin deficiency.
- Connective tissue diseases.
- Thyroid disease: previous treatment with radioiodine.
- Diseases associated with pernicious anemia (e.g., vitiligo, diabetes mellitus, thyroiditis).
- Jaundice (e.g., alcohol abuse, chronic liver disease, hemolysis).

Drug history

A particularly detailed drug history is important as often drugs can cause or exacerbate anemia. Drugs can cause anemia in many ways. For example:
- Blood loss (aspirin or NSAIDs).
- Hemolysis: immune-mediated (e.g., quinidine, methyldopa), glucose-6-phosphate dehydrogenase (G6PD) deficiency (e.g., antimalarials, dapsone).
- Aplasia: cytotoxic chemotherapy, idiopathic (e.g., sulfonamides).

- Megaloblastic anemia: phenytoin, dihydrofolate reductase inhibitors (trimethoprim, methotrexate).
- Sideroblastic anemia (isoniazid).

Family history

Consider the possibility of an inherited hemolytic anemia (especially in the appropriate ethnic group). For example:
- Sickle cell anemia: especially in sub-Saharan Africans and malarial areas.
- Thalassemia: especially in those from the Mediterranean, Middle East, India, Southeast Asia.
- Hereditary spherocytosis: northern Europeans.
- G6PD deficiency: in people from West Africa, Mediterranean, Middle East, Southeast Asia.

Social history

Focus on the diet, especially if there is iron, folate, or vitamin B_{12} deficiency.

History of risk-taking behavior

Alcohol can cause anemia in many ways.

Review of systems

As the cause of anemia is often multifactorial, the ROS is often fruitful. In particular, consider causes of chronic blood loss (e.g., dyspepsia, melena, menorrhagia) and symptoms suggestive of systemic disease (e.g., weight loss, fevers, sweats).

If a particular cause of anemia is suspected, specific questions relating to that system should be asked in detail.

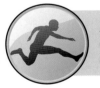 Anemia is often multifactorial, so a detailed history is essential to elucidate different components. A diagnosis of iron deficiency is inadequate. The underlying cause for the deficiency must be found. Always ask about the use of aspirin or NSAIDs.

Acute gastrointestinal bleeding

Presenting complaint

Typical presentations include vomiting blood (hematemesis), dyspepsia, abdominal pain, and "tarry black stools," which are very often smelly (melena).

History of present illness

Acute GI bleeding is a medical emergency and should be assessed via the ABC approach.

The most common causes of acute upper gastrointestinal (GI) bleeding include the following (those with an asterisk are the most common):
- Gastric ulcer.*
- Duodenal ulcer.*
- Gastric erosions and gastritis.*
- Mallory–Weiss syndrome.
- Esophageal varices.
- Hemorrhagic peptic esophagitis.
- Gastric carcinoma (rarely presents with an acute GI bleed).
- Hereditary hemorrhagic telangiectasia (rare).

Acute lower gastrointestinal bleeding may be due to:
- Bleeding hemorrhoids.
- Diverticulosis.

Ask questions about hemodynamic stability:
- Faintness and loss of consciousness.
- Sweating.
- Palpitations.
- Confusion.

The presence of melena indicates that the source of blood loss is probably proximal to and including the cecum. It is not enough to accept a history of melena. A digital rectal examination must be performed to positively confirm or refute this.

Obtain a detailed history, focusing on symptoms referable to the gastrointestinal tract. Ask specifically about abdominal pain, dyspepsia and heartburn, vomiting and nausea, weight loss, and early satiety.

Ask about the duration of symptoms. It is worth inquiring whether the patient has experienced any symptoms suggestive of anemia (e.g., lethargy, angina, palpitations, unexplained fatigue).

There may be a periodicity and relationship to food or identifiable precipitating events, for example, an alcoholic binge, vomiting (e.g., Mallory–Weiss syndrome, pyloric stenosis).

Past medical history

Ask about pre-existing GI tract pathologies and investigations (e.g., endoscopy, barium swallow). Liver disease or jaundice may suggest gastritis or esophageal varices in the presence of portal hypertension.

Drug history

Ask specifically about:
- Aspirin and NSAIDs (common causes of gastritis).
- Steroids (may exacerbate pre-existing ulcer).
- Use of antacids, histamine H_2 blockers, proton pump inhibitors.

Family history

Patients with peptic ulceration often have a positive family history.

History of risk-taking behavior

Cigarettes are associated with peptic ulceration. Alcohol is strongly associated with liver disease and gastritis. Binge drinkers may have been vomiting and have produced Mallory–Weiss tears.

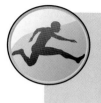

The underlying cause of the bleed is often indicated from the history, but subsequent confirmation by endoscopy is almost invariably indicated.

Change in bowel habit

Presenting complaint

Patients may present with either a change in normal stool frequency or a change in the nature of the stool.

History of present illness

The main conditions producing a change in bowel habit are illustrated in Fig. 6.11. Find out the patient's normal pattern of bowel movements. A normal pattern varies from one stool every three days to three stools per day. Inquire specifically about the frequency of stools, and do not accept terms such as "diarrhea" or "constipation" without clarification.

Ask about the duration of symptoms. A very short history of a few hours is likely to indicate an infective etiology, whereas altered bowel habit for many years is more likely to indicate irritable bowel disorder in a young patient. Ask specifically about weight loss, anorexia, fatigue, and their onset.

Associated abdominal pain may suggest an anatomical site of pathology (e.g., left iliac fossa pain is common with disease of the sigmoid colon).

Inquire about the presence of blood in the stool. The color and relationship to the stool may reveal its origin, as follows:

- Bright-red blood on the surface of the stool occurs with rectosigmoid lesions (e.g., polyp, carcinoma) or hemorrhoids.
- Red blood mixed with the stool is a feature of colorectal lesions (e.g., polyp, carcinoma, inflammatory bowel disease, diverticular disease).
- Altered blood or clots almost always imply significant pathology (e.g., colorectal lesion such as polyp, carcinoma, inflammatory bowel disease, diverticular disease).

Inquire about the presence of mucus or slime in the stool (Fig. 6.12). If it is associated with blood, the most likely causes are inflammatory bowel disease or colorectal carcinoma. If mucus or slime occurs in isolation, irritable bowel syndrome may also be a cause.

Finally, ask about other characteristics of the stool. For example:

- Stools of reduced caliber occur in low strictures.
- Fatty, floating, difficult to flush, offensive stools suggest steatorrhea.
- Pellet-like or "stringy" stools occur in diverticular disease or irritable bowel syndrome.

Causes of change in bowel habit	
Condition	Features
colorectal carcinoma	weight loss; chronic history; blood in the stool
inflammatory bowel disease	Crohn's disease; ulcerative colitis; ask about systemic manifestations (e.g., arthropathy, oral ulcers, weight loss, etc.)
diverticular disease	very common; older patients; hard to diagnose from the history and examination alone
colonic polyps	may have mucoid discharge
infective colitis	usually acute, explosive history
irritable bowel syndrome	colicky abdominal pain; bloating; mucus; related to stress; absence of any sinister features in the history; very common

Fig. 6.11 Causes of change in bowel habit. Asterisks indicate the more common causes.

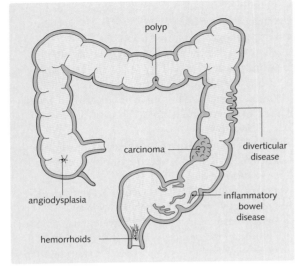

Fig. 6.12 Potential sources of rectal bleeding.

Causes of dysphagia in the esophagus	
Type of lesion	Example
obstruction within the lumen	carcinoma of the esophagus; peptic stricture; foreign body; lower esophageal ring
extrinsic compression of the esophagus	mediastinal lymphadenopathy
motility disorder of the esophagus	achalasia of the esophagus; esophageal spasm, scleroderma; Chagas' disease; diabetic autonomic neuropathy

Fig. 6.13 Causes of dysphagia in the esophagus.

History of risk-taking behavior

If there is unexplained diarrhea, consider the patient's risk factors for HIV infection.

Past medical history

A detailed history is essential, but previous surgical or medical problems may elucidate the cause of the change in bowel habit. For example:

- Previous colonic polyps, abdominal surgery.
- Thyroid disease.
- Malabsorption syndromes (e.g., pancreatitis).
- Diabetes mellitus (autonomic neuropathy).

Drug history

Many drugs can cause a change in bowel habit. For example:

- Constipation: opiates, anticholinergic agents, tricyclic antidepressants.
- Diarrhea: thyroxine, laxative abuse, magnesium salts, broad-spectrum antibiotics (specifically consider pseudomembranous colitis).

Family history

Some diseases causing a change in bowel habit have a genetic component. For example:

- Familial adenomatous polyposis.
- Inflammatory bowel disease.
- Carcinoma of the bowel.

Social history

Ask about foreign travel for amebiasis, giardiasis, and typhoid.

Dysphagia

History of present illness

Dysphagia refers either to difficulty in swallowing or pain on swallowing. Although the cause usually requires specific investigations (e.g., barium swallow, endoscopy, and biopsy), the history is important in directing these investigations. The main causes of dysphagia are indicated in Fig. 6.13.

What does the patient mean by dysphagia?

It is important to clarify exactly what patients mean when they say that they have difficulty in swallowing. It is not acceptable to write "Patient complains of dysphagia" in the medical notes.

True dysphagia almost always indicates the presence of an organic lesion. It is important to distinguish dysphagia from "globus hystericus" (the sensation of a lump or fullness in the throat associated with chronic anxiety states).

How bad is the dysphagia?

Try to assess the functional impact. Dysphagia often progresses from solid food to soft food and liquid. Ask the patient to describe exactly which foods cause difficulty. Ascertain whether there is complete obstruction (e.g., regurgitation immediately after attempting to swallow food, vomiting).

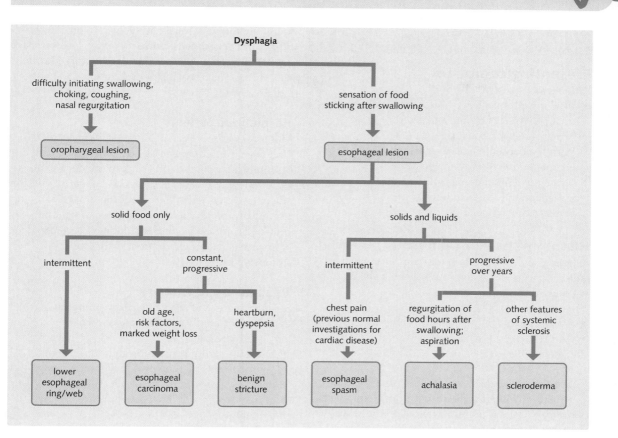

Fig. 6.14 Features from the history to aid the differential diagnosis of dysphagia.

 Weight loss is a useful indicator of a serious underlying organic disorder and should always be asked about specifically.

Duration and time course of symptoms

Ask patients how long they have had difficulty swallowing.

- Malignancy often presents over weeks or months and is typically progressive.
- An esophageal ring may present over a similar time course but produces a more intermittent pattern.
- Other causes may be present for years without any obvious systemic disturbance (e.g., globus hystericus).

Clues to underlying pathology

Specifically inquire about previous dyspepsia, proven peptic ulcer disease, or reflux. Ask about symptoms of heartburn such as acid taste in the mouth, retrosternal burning, relationship to posture. These symptoms suggest the presence of a benign esophageal stricture.

Look for risk factors for esophageal cancer such as:
- Cigarette smoking.
- Barrett's esophagus.
- Old age.
- Heavy alcohol use.
- Significant weight loss.

Dysphagia to solid foods alone suggests a mechanical obstruction, dysphagia to liquids to a greater extent than solids suggests a neuromuscular cause.

Ask the patient where the food appears to get stuck. Symptoms such as difficulty initiating swallowing, coughing, choking, or nasal regurgitation suggest an oropharyngeal pathology. A sensation of food sticking after swallowing suggests an esophageal lesion (Fig. 6.14).

Acute renal failure

Presenting complaint

Patients may present in various ways:

- With symptoms directly referable to the renal tract (relatively rare presentation) (e.g., with hematuria, flank pain).
- With the consequences of renal failure (e.g., edema, uremic symptoms, hypertension).
- As an incidental finding from laboratory investigation (e.g., biochemical profile from investigation of other disease).

History of present illness

Ask specifically about uremic symptoms, which may indicate the need for hemodialysis. Ask about:

- Nausea, vomiting.
- Anorexia.
- Malaise, lethargy.
- Pruritus.
- Hiccupping.

Note that many of these symptoms are nonspecific.

Specifically inquire about symptoms referable to the urinary tract as these may indicate the etiology of the renal dysfunction. For example:

- Prostatism: may suggest outflow obstruction.
- Hematuria: inquire specifically about the color if hematuria is present (often described as "like cola" in glomerulonephritis; bright red usually implies lower urinary tract bleeding).
- Dysuria, frequency (may suggest infective etiology).
- Oliguria or anuria (may suggest prerenal disease or severe renal failure).

Complications of renal failure

These may be present. For example:

- Peripheral edema.
- Hypertension.
- Dyspnea due to pulmonary edema.

Duration of disease

It is often difficult to elicit the duration of the disease as often the symptoms begin insidiously and are usually very nonspecific. Clues may be obtained by asking specifically about, for example, change in weight or fatigue. Ask "When did you last feel completely well?" and "Have you been more tired than usual lately?" This may date the onset of renal failure, but usually renal pathology remains clinically silent until decompensation occurs or it is discovered incidentally. However, a meticulous history may help date the original renal insult in different circumstances.

Hospitalized patients

Most cases of acute renal failure occur in hospital. Create a flowchart of the blood results (especially biochemical profile) dating back to the decline in renal function. It is usually possible to identify within one or two days when the creatinine started to rise. At this point, focus on events that might have provided a critical insult to the kidneys (e.g., period of hypotension or dehydration, toxic levels of aminoglycosides, coexisting infection).

Past medical history

Since the causes of renal failure are numerous, detailed past medical history is essential. In particular, consider:

- Diabetes mellitus: duration and presence of neuropathy or retinopathy, which are almost invariably associated with diabetic nephropathy.
- Hypertension: did it predate or postdate renal dysfunction?
- Risk factors for renovascular disease, such as claudication, aortic aneurysm, ischemic heart disease, hypercholesterolemia.
- Childhood enuresis or frequent urinary tract infections, suggesting reflux nephropathy.
- Renal stones or colic.
- Autoimmune diseases, such as systemic lupus erythematosus (SLE), rheumatoid arthritis, scleroderma.
- Jaundice (e.g., hepatitis B, hepatitis C-associated glomerulopathy, leptospirosis, hepatorenal syndrome).
- Recent infections, such as postinfectious glomerulonephritis, presentation of IgA nephropathy with hematuria following a sore throat.

Drug history

Again a detailed drug history is essential. Very often, drugs have precipitated the renal failure. Remember to ask about over-the-counter medication and herbal remedies.

Drugs may precipitate renal failure by various mechanisms (Fig. 6.15). Other drugs must be used with caution in renal failure. For example:

Mechanisms of drug-induced renal dysfunction

Pathology	Drugs
decreased renal perfusion	diuretics* (hypovolemia); NSAIDs* (also cause interstitial nephritis, hyperkalemia, and rarely papillary necrosis)
decreased glomerular filtration pressure	ACE inhibitors*
nephrotic syndrome	gold; penicillamine
acute tubular necrosis	aminoglycosides* (especially if toxic drug levels); antibiotics (e.g., cephalosporins); contrast agents (especially in diabetics); chemotherapy (e.g., cisplatin)
interstitial nephritis	NSAIDs*; antibiotics* (e.g., penicillin, sulfonamides)
renal stones	cytotoxic agents (especially in lymphoma)
electrolyte disturbances	diuretics* (especially hypokalemia); renal tubular acidosis (acetazolamide); inappropriate ADH secretion (carbamazepine, chlorpropamide); hyperkalemia (NSAIDs, ACE inhibitors, diuretics acting on distal tubule)
retroperitoneal fibrosis	methysergide

Fig. 6.15 Mechanisms of drug-induced renal dysfunction. Asterisks indicate the more commonly implicated drugs. (ACE, angiotensin-converting enzyme; ADH, antidiuretic hormone; NSAID, nonsteroidal anti-inflamatory drug.)

- Renally excreted drugs (aminoglycosides).
- If there is an accumulation of metabolites due to failure of clearance (opiates).

Family history
Consider inherited conditions (e.g., polycystic kidneys, Alport's syndrome).

Social history
It is essential to obtain as much background information as possible to assess normal functional capacity. The social history should include travel and ethnic origin. Many forms of glomerulonephritis demonstrate great geographical variation (e.g., IgA nephropathy is more common in Caucasians, SLE is more common in African-Americans).

History of risk-taking behavior
- Cigarette smoking (renovascular disease).
- Alcohol (hepatorenal disease).
- Risk factors for HIV and hepatitis B and C (glomerulonephritis, hepatorenal disease).

Review of systems
Vital information may be omitted if the ROS is not performed. In particular, consider:

- Symptoms suggestive of autoimmune etiology: skin rash, arthralgia, myalgia, alopecia, early morning stiffness.
- Fevers: any infective or inflammatory disease.

Chronic renal failure

Presenting complaint
It is assumed that the patient will already be on dialysis or is being reviewed in the predialysis clinic and that the cause of renal disease has already been investigated (see previous section).

History of present illness
Dialysis
Assess symptoms indicative of inadequate dialysis or need to commence dialysis:
- Anorexia.
- Nausea, vomiting.
- Fatigue, malaise.
- Confusion, drowsiness.

Although many of these symptoms are nonspecific, if no other cause is found, assume that they represent uremia.

Features of peritoneal dialysis and hemodialysis to elicit from the history		
Parameter	Peritoneal dialysis	Hemodialysis
mode of dialysis	continuous ambulatory peritoneal dialysis (CAPD); automated peritoneal dialysis (APD)	hospital hemodialysis; home hemodialysis
dialysis dose	number and type of bags (e.g., "light/heavy"); volume of fluid (typically 2 L)	hours on dialysis; frequency (typically 4 hours three times weekly)
access	PD exit site	arteriovenous (AV) fistula; temporary catheter (e.g., "vascath"); AV shunt
complications of dialysis	peritonitis; exit site and tunnel infections	dialysis dysequilibrium; hypotensive episodes; difficulty needing fistula; exit site infections: vascular stenosis

Fig. 6.16 Features of peritoneal dialysis (PD) and hemodialysis (HD).

Dialysis-related problems

Dialysis is associated with a number of specific problems or issues, which need to be considered, whether the form of dialysis is peritoneal dialysis or hemodialysis. Review the mechanics and complications of dialysis (Fig. 6.16).

Fluid balance

There are many common problems of chronic renal failure, and these should always be addressed. Review fluid balance, which is central to the management. It is essential to ask about the following:

- Does the patient have a target "dry" weight? Fluctuations from this weight in the short term usually indicate fluid shifts.
- Urine output and daily fluid restriction, which is usually 500 mL more than daily urine output.
- Interdialysis weight gains. Large gains may indicate poor compliance and understanding of self-management.

Anemia

Review symptoms (e.g., dyspnea, lethargy, decreased exercise tolerance). Many patients will be taking recombinant erythropoietin. Always specifically inquire about and record:

- The dose.
- Side effects (e.g., hypertension, hyperkalemia).
- Reasons for lack of response to erythropoietin (e.g., iron deficiency, intercurrent infection, hyperparathyroidism).

Renal osteodystrophy

Renal osteodystrophy is a common problem of chronic renal failure and should be explored. From the notes and patient account review:

- Calcium and phosphate balance.
- Diet.
- Calcium carbonate dose.
- Biochemical evidence for hyperparathyroidism.

Transplant status

Review plans for discharging the patient from this form of dialysis. In particular, consider (at every visit) the appropriateness for transplantation, taking into account the patient's wishes and knowledge. Review intercurrent medical issues that may preclude transplantation, such as age, infection, malignancy, severe vascular disease, untreated ischemic heart disease, active peptic ulceration.

Blood pressure control

Review the documentary evidence of blood pressure measurements—for example, from dialysis charts or recordings made at home (before erythropoietin dosing) or by the primary care physician.

Past medical history

This is usually well known. Do not forget the original cause of the renal failure!

Drug history

A meticulous drug history is essential. Very often the patient will have a long list of medications. Inquire specifically about:

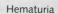

- Antihypertensive agents.
- Erythropoietin (see above).
- Phosphate binders and vitamin D.
- Iron supplements.
- Over-the-counter medication.

Consider drugs to be used with caution in renal failure (see "Acute renal failure").

Social history
A detailed assessment should be made, especially in the predialysis patient, when considering whether dialysis would be appropriate, and if so, which form.
If considering hemodialysis:
- Will transport be needed to the hospital?

If considering chronic ambulatory peritoneal dialysis (CAPD):
- Does the patient have space at home to store boxes containing peritoneal dialysis fluid?
- Does the patient have the manual dexterity needed to change bags?
- Does the patient have the motivation and intelligence to manage the care so that there is not an undue risk for developing peritonitis or site infections?
- Is the patient obese?

Review the patient's nutrition and diet. This is often specialized, and referral to a renal dietician is indicated.

Review of systems
This is particularly important because patients are often multisymptomatic and renal failure is associated with so many other diseases (e.g., ischemic heart disease, arthritis, gastrointestinal bleeding).

Chronic renal failure results in mutisystem dysfunction. Assessment needs to be detailed. It is pointless to rush. Always allow enough time. In predialysis patients, check that adequate plans have been made for the initiation of dialysis so that the transition can be as smooth as possible. Consider patient education, mode of intended dialysis, access for dialysis, and estimated time to dialysis initiation.

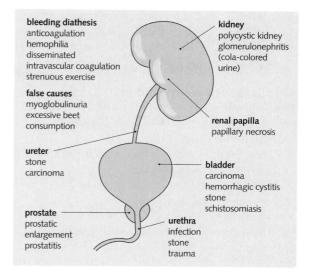

Fig. 6.17 Some causes of hematuria.

Hematuria

History of present illness
Hematuria is a common symptom and may be due to a wide variety of pathologies (Fig. 6.17). Take a full history of the presenting symptom.

Ascertain that true hematuria is present
Some patients with uterine bleeding mistakenly believe that they have hematuria.

Duration
Note whether the hematuria is an acute presentation or has been present for many years or months.

Nature
A small amount of blood produces visible discoloration of the urine. Try to establish how much blood is present in the urine. It may be helpful to ask:
- "Are there any blood clots in your urine?"
- "Is your urine bright red or stained like blackcurrant juice?'"
- "Does your urine appear cloudy or like cola?" (glomerulonephritis).

The timing of blood during the urinary stream may provide a clue to the origin of bleeding. For example:
- Bleeding at the start of the urinary stream suggests a urethral lesion.

- Bleeding through the whole stream suggests a source in the bladder or higher in the urinary tract.
- Bleeding at the end of the urinary stream suggests a source in the lower bladder.

Associated urinary symptoms

Other symptoms referable to the urinary tract often provide useful clues to the cause of hematuria. Specifically ask about:
- Dysuria and frequency with small quantities of urine (urinary tract infection).
- The above symptoms in association with fever and flank pain suggest pyelonephritis.
- Colicky flank pain is indicative of renal stones.
- Symptoms of renal disease such as ankle swelling or uremic symptoms.
- Terminal dribbling, hesitancy, and poor stream are common in prostatic obstruction.

Past medical history

A detailed past medical history is important. In particular, ask about:
- Previous renal disease.
- Abdominal trauma (e.g., renal capsular tear).

- Renal stones or previous episodes of colic.
- Previous cystoscopies.
- Prostatectomy (in men).
- Sickle cell anemia (papillary necrosis).

Drug history

Some drugs may aggravate or cause hematuria. For example:
- Cyclophosphamide (hemorrhagic cystitis, carcinoma of the bladder).
- Warfarin (bleeding diathesis).
- Analgesic abuse (papillary necrosis).

Family history

Many renal diseases have a familial tendency. For example:
- Polycystic kidney disease (adult variety is autosomal dominant).
- Alport's syndrome (X-linked recessive). Ask about deafness.
- IgA nephropathy. Ask about the relationship of macroscopic hematuria to infections.
- Sickle cell anemia.

7. Presenting Problems: Nervous System

Overview

Nervous system disease presents with a full range of symptoms ranging from loss of consciousness through loss of motor or sensory function to back pain, headache, and chronic pain. As a subjective symptom without distinct physical examination findings, pain challenges the clinician to take a careful history and differentiate between organic and functional disease.

The unconscious patient

History of present illness

The history is especially important in the evaluation of the unconscious patient, even though it may not come from the patient. Obtain the history from relatives or friends, the ambulance crew, or police, if appropriate. Try to establish the following.

Time of onset of unconsciousness

Who found the patient unconscious and when? When was the patient last seen conscious? Where was the patient found?

Duration of illness preceding unconsciousness

Had the patient been well before being found unconscious? Was the illness sudden (minutes), gradual (hours), or chronic (days to weeks)?

Nature of the preceding illness

It is helpful to consider the differential diagnosis, so that questions can be more focused (Fig. 7.1).

Past medical history

Obtain a full history. There may have been previous episodes. Inquire specifically about:
- Diabetes mellitus (hypoglycemia, hyperglycemic coma).
- Risk factors for cerebrovascular disease (stroke).
- Epilepsy and other neurological disorders.
- Head trauma, no matter how mild and how much in the past; a subdural hematoma may be preceded by a history of a trivial head injury, especially in the elderly.
- Preceding headaches (e.g., meningitis, intracranial mass lesion, subarachnoid hemorrhage).
- Renal failure.
- Liver failure.
- Vomiting.

Drug history

Consider all drugs that may depress the conscious level if taken in therapeutic or toxic amounts. Remember to ask about analgesic agents and psychotropic medication.

History of risk-taking behavior

This is particularly important, especially in younger patients. Ask specifically about:
- Alcohol (very important).
- Drugs of abuse (very important).
- Possible reasons for deliberate self-harm.

Do not underestimate the importance of the history, even if the patient cannot provide one directly. The differential diagnosis is broad, but can usually be narrowed down with the aid of a well-taken history from a third party. Detailed history taking often needs to be deferred until appropriate resuscitation or stabilization has been carried out.

Blackouts

History of present illness

A common problem for admitting medical teams is the investigation of a patient who has had a blackout. The history is central to the diagnosis. It is imperative to find out what the patient means by the term "blackout." Follow the usual systematic approach to investigate circumstances of the blackout. It is helpful to consider the differential diagnosis of blackouts (Fig. 7.2).

Clues from the history on the underlying cause of unconsciousness	
Description	**Indications**

vascular*
   subarachnoid hemorrhage*
   intracerebral bleed*,
   massive infarction*,
   brainstem stroke*
	preceding headache; sudden onset; often young adult; may have had "herald bleed" risk factors for cerebrovascular disease (hypertension, diabetes mellitus (DM), ischemic heart disease, age, family history, etc.)

metabolic*
   DM*
 	
   drugs and toxins*
   hypoxia,
   hyponatremia,
   hypothyroidsm*,
   uremia,
   hepatic encephalopathy
	hyperosmolar coma (type II DM); diabetic ketoacidosis (type I—may be presenting feature of disease); hypoglycemia alcohol*; sedative drugs (opiates, benzodiazepines, barbiturates, etc.) often present nonspecifically

sepsis
   generalized,
   meningoencephalitis,
   brain abscess
	usually preceding illness; ask about rash, photophobia, fevers, headache, vomiting, etc.

subdural*/extradural hematoma	may be history of trauma (often absent)
postictal	may find bottle of antiepileptic tablets
intracranial mass lesion	ask about features of raised intracranial pressure (e.g., increasing morning headache, vomiting, developing focal neurological problems)
factitious/hysteria	often unusual presentation; past psychiatric history

Fig. 7.1 Clues from the history on the underlying cause of unconsciousness. Asterisks indicate the more common causes. DM, diabetes mellitus.

Differential diagnosis of blackouts

epilepsy*

decreased cerebral perfusion
vasovagal episode*; cardiac disturbances* (e.g., arrhythmia, aortic stenosis, ischemia); postural hypotension*; TIA (especially in posterior circulation); micturition syncope (decreased venous return during breath holding); cough syncope (decreased venous return); carotid sinus hypersensitivity

metabolic disturbances
hypoglycemia; hypocalcemia

psychological
panic attacks*; hyperventilation*; factitious

drugs
alcohol*; recreational drugs of abuse; prescribed medication (e.g., decreased threshold for epileptic seizure, sedative, beta-blockers provoking profound bradycardia, etc.)

Fig. 7.2 Differential diagnosis of blackouts. TIA, transient ischemic attack.

Investigate the episode chronologically. Find out what the patient was doing immediately before blacking out, whether the patient had any warning symptoms, and how the patient felt immediately after regaining consciousness (Fig. 7.3).

Did anyone witness the episode?

This is probably the most useful piece of information. If so, ask specifically about:
- How long the blackout lasted (seconds, minutes, or hours).
- What was the patient doing during the episode? (e.g., lying still, shaking, appearing confused, purposeful movements).
- The presence of any incontinence or shaking to suggest an epileptic fit.
- Did anyone feel the pulse either during or immediately after the blackout? A normal pulse during the blackout would exclude an arrhythmia. Remember to evaluate the competence of the person who felt the pulse.

Clues from the history on the underlying pathology responsible for an episode of loss of consciousness	
Clues from the history	**Possible underlying cause of blackout**

"What were you doing immediately before blacking out?"
  standing up quickly
  turning head sharply
  trauma
  completely at rest
  standing still in hot environment
	
	postural hypotension
	cervical spondylosis (occlusion of vertebral artery)
	subdural hematoma; extradural hematoma; contusion injury
	arrhythmia; cerebrovascular disease, etc.
	vasovagal

"Did you have any warning that you were going to blackout?"
  aura
  palpitations, chest pain
  lightheadedness
  sweating, hunger
	
	epileptic seizure
	cardiogenic; panic attack
	vasovagal, etc.
	hypoglycemia

Fig. 7.3 Clues from the history on the underlying pathology responsible for an episode of loss of consciousness.

Try to establish whether the episode was a true syncopal attack (loss of consciousness and motor tone) or just a period of lightheadedness. Very often people say that they have blacked out when they do not completely lose consciousness: ask, for example, "Did you lose any time?," "Were you out cold?"

Inquire about the immediate period following recovery of consciousness. Symptoms at this stage may give clues to the precipitating event. For example:

- Immediate recovery (vasovagal).
- Confusion and disorientation (e.g., postictal).
- Weakness: Todd's paralysis, transient ischemic attack (TIA).

Past medical history

Ask about previous blackouts and investigations performed. Consider clues from the past history that may increase the probability of certain underlying problems. For example:

- Risk factors for epilepsy (e.g., head injury, cerebrovascular disease, meningitis).
- Cardiac diseases.
- Diabetes mellitus: inquire about medication, diabetic control, and previous episodes of hypoglycemia.

Drug history

A full drug history is essential. In particular, consider:
- Recent changes to prescribed drugs.

- Negative chronotropic and inotropic agents (e.g., beta-blockers).
- Drugs likely to cause arrhythmias (e.g., tricyclic antidepressants, theophylline).
- Insulin (hypoglycemia).
- Antihypertensive agents (postural hypotension).
- Illicit drug use.

Social history

Investigate whether the home environment is safe for someone who may blackout unexpectedly (e.g., are there any caregivers at home?). The patient's lifestyle may suggest underlying risks for a blackout (e.g., alcohol consumption, unusual stresses at home or work).

Review of systems

Blackouts may result from a wide range of pathologies, so a review of systems may reveal unexpected pathology. Focus on the cardiovascular, neurological, metabolic, and musculoskeletal systems.

The key to diagnosing the cause of a blackout is a well-taken history. The most useful information comes from an eyewitness account.

Features of different types of headache

Headache	Characteristics
tension headache	most common recurrent headache, typically described as "throbbing," "pressure," etc. often identifiable precipitating factor (e.g., stress, depression)
migraine	common cause of recurrent headache; usually presents in young adults; prodrome—often visual (e.g., scotomata, teichopsia), tingling, etc.; headache—often starts unilaterally; associated symptoms (e.g., nausea, vomiting, photophobia, etc.)
subarachnoid hemorrhage	may have had "herald bleed" with milder "subclinical" episodes; typically sudden onset "like a hammer hitting the back of my head"; may have associated neurological deficit or decreased level of consciousness
hangover	previous alcohol consumption; associated nausea
meningitis	photophobia; neck stiffness; fever; rash
raised intracranial pressure	usually subacute onset; relentless; present on waking; aggravated by coughing, sneezing, stooping, associated nausea
temporal arteritis	pain over superficial temporal arteries, especially on touching area (e.g., combing hair); may have associated malaise, proximal muscle weakness and stiffness, and visual loss; usually older than 60 years

Fig. 7.4 Features of different types of headache.

Headache

History of the present illness

Consider the following common causes of single and recurrent headaches:

- Tension headache (by far the most common).
- Migraine (common).
- Hangover (apparent from the history).
- Subarachnoid hemorrhage (rare, but consider for any sudden-onset headache).
- Meningitis, encephalitis.
- Raised intracranial pressure (e.g., tumor, hydrocephalus).
- Temporal arteritis.

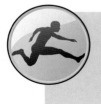

20% of headaches presenting in the ED are subarachnoid hemorrhages; the most common mistake is to diagnose them as migraine.

Obtain a detailed history about the frequency of headaches. For example, recurrent headaches are typically tension headaches or migraine, while a headache every morning can be due to raised intracranial pressure associated with a tumor.

For any new-onset headache, always ask specifically about photophobia, neck stiffness, rash, fever, and vomiting.

Obtain information about the onset, nature, and location of headache. It is often possible to identify the cause of a headache from these parameters (Figs. 7.4 and 7.5).

Past medical history

Ask specifically about previous malignancy if raised intracranial pressure is suspected.

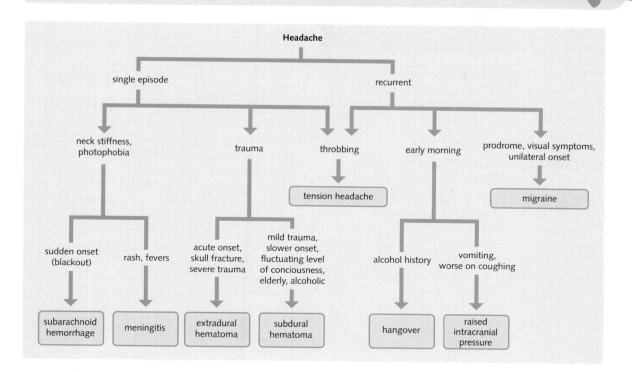

Fig. 7.5 Differential diagnosis of headache.

Drug history

Ask about medication taken to relieve symptoms and efficacy. It is often hard to assess the severity of headache as people can rarely give a quantitative description. It may be worth asking, "If 0 is no pain and 10 is the worst headache you have ever had, what score would you give this pain?" Ask all women about the use of oral contraceptives (may precipitate or worsen migraine particularly in the pill-free week).

Social history and history of risk-taking behavior

For recurrent headaches, it is essential to ask about stresses (e.g., at home and work) that may be precipitating chronic nonspecific headaches. The patient's alcohol history is also relevant. Eliciting the patient's ideas and concerns about the headache is especially important as many are worried about serious pathology (e.g., brain tumor or stroke).

Headache is a universal condition. The principal aim is to distinguish nonserious benign headaches from those that may represent serious underlying pathology needing further investigation so that appropriate reassurance can be given. Always consider headaches representing serious disease. Alarm words may include:
- Scalp tenderness, proximal limb stiffness (temporal arteritis).
- Rash, fever, photophobia, neck stiffness (meningitis).
- Sudden-onset occipital headache (subarachnoid hemorrhage).
- Early morning headache, nausea (raised intracranial pressure).

Epileptic seizure

Presenting complaint

Epilepsy may present as an unwitnessed blackout (single or recurrent) or as an eyewitness account of a seizure. More rarely it may present with behavioral changes.

History of present illness

Start with the patient's own recollection of the event, recording the following chronologically.

Prodrome

Ask "Did you have any warning that you were going to blackout?" Typical auras include sensations that the patient may find difficult to describe, including strange thoughts, emotions, or hallucinations (e.g., smell, taste, vision). They often follow a predictable course for the individual patient.

Seizure

Ask "Tell me what you remember about the attack?" and "Did you blackout and lose consciousness?" The answers to these questions may help distinguish between generalized and partial seizures. If the patient was conscious during the episode, ask him or her to describe exactly what happened. If the patient has experienced a partial seizure, the symptoms are often characteristic of the site of epileptic focus. For example:
- Jacksonian motor seizures.
- Temporal lobe epilepsy (e.g., déjà vu, jamais vu, hallucinations of smell or taste).

It is usually possible to distinguish partial seizures, generalized seizures, and partial seizures with secondary generalization.

Postical period

Ask "How did you feel when you came around?" It is usual to experience a headache, fuzziness, lethargy, confusion, and nonspecific malaise. A focal weakness may be present for up to 24 hours (Todd's paralysis).

Obtain an eyewitness account if possible. This is invaluable and can provide diagnostic information.

If the episode was a single blackout, the most common difficulty is distinguishing between epilepsy and syncope. Look for an identifiable precipitant for syncope (e.g., emotional stress, prolonged standing, cough, micturition syncope), gradual onset and recovery, and pallor and flaccidity during the episode. Be aware that a convulsion or urinary incontinence rarely occurs during syncopal episodes.

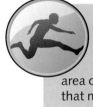 Generalized seizures imply widespread abnormal electrical activity in the brain, while partial seizures imply a discrete area of abnormal electrical activity that may or may not spread.

On the basis of the history, try to decide on the type of epilepsy (Fig. 7.6). If the patient has had multiple seizures, ask about seizure control (i.e.,

Historical features of different types of epilepsy	
generalized seizures	
tonic–clonic seizure (grand mal)*	most commonly perceived form of epilepsy—"convulsions"
absence seizures (petit mal)*	especially in childhood; brief (few seconds) loss of consciousness; no fall; no convulsion
myoclonic seizures	especially in childhood; usually symmetrical
tonic seizures	especially in childhood; loss of consciousness; usually underlying organic brain disease
akinetic seizures	no prodrome ("drop attacks")
partial seizures	
simple partial seizures*	remains fully conscious during attack (e.g., jacksonian seizure)
complex partial seizures*	originates in the temporal lobe; often complex sensory hallucinations, déjà vu, jamais vu, lip smacking, chewing, behavioral disturbances, etc.
partial seizure with secondary generalization*	as above, but progresses to tonic–clonic seizure

Fig. 7.6 The history often reveals the type of epilepsy. Asterisks indicate the more common causes.

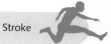

frequency of seizures, duration of seizures). Ask about precipitating factors (e.g., flickering lights).

Past medical history
Consider possible underlying causes of fits (Fig. 7.7).

Drug history
Ask about drugs used to control epilepsy and their side effects (e.g., phenytoin, sodium valproate, carbamazepine). Ask specifically about symptoms suggestive of overdose (e.g., drowsiness, ataxia, slurred speech). Review adherence, especially if there is evidence of poor seizure control, and consider the need to check drug levels (phenytoin has a narrow therapeutic index).

Consider medication that may:
- Interact with anticonvulsants (e.g., oral contraceptives, warfarin).
- Lower the seizure threshold (e.g., phenothiazines, tricyclic antidepressants, amphetamines).

Family history
In younger patients, there is often a positive family history.

Social history and history of risk-taking behavior
There are multiple social issues surrounding epilepsy. Often patients feel stigmatized and socially isolated. School performance is often poor. The reasons for this should be explored (e.g., poorly controlled seizures, drug intoxication, social isolation and bullying, underlying brain disease). Parents are often understandably overprotective. Consider sensible restrictions on activities for children while allowing a full social life (e.g., avoiding known precipitants such as strobe lighting at discos, bathing in a locked bathroom, or dangerous sports such as rock climbing).

Consider the restrictions on driving. This may affect the decision to start withdrawing medication in patients with well-controlled disease if driving is particularly important to them.

Review occupational problems (e.g., use of dangerous machinery, employers who do not understand the disease).

In common with many other neurological events, try to obtain a good eyewitness account of a typical episode as very often the patient is asymptomatic and has no physical signs on presentation to a doctor.

Underlying pathology causing seizures
cerebrovascular disease*
most common cause in older age group; risk factors (e.g., hypertension, smoking, ischemic heart disease, diabetes mellitus, etc.)
alcohol and drug withdrawal*
drugs*
for example tricyclic antidepressants, phenothiazines, amphetamines, etc.
head injury and neurosurgery
tumors
encephalitis
degenerative brain disease
metabolic disorders
for example hypoglycemia, hyponatremia, hypocalcemia, uremia, liver failure, etc.
fever
NB febrile convulsions are not epilepsy

Fig. 7.7 Underlying pathology responsible for epileptic seizures can often be identified. Asterisks indicate the more common causes.

Stroke

Strokes are common and take up large amounts of healthcare resources. They are the third most common cause of death in the developed world. 80% of all strokes are embolic events, and 10% of people with infarcts will die within 30 days. (See Gubitz & Sandercock, *Br Med J* **320**, 692–6.)

History of the present illness
Establish that the described event is a stroke. It is usually obvious from the history that a stroke has occurred. Try to work out where in the cerebral circulation the stroke has occurred as this has prognostic value (see Figs. 7.8 and 7.9).

Fig. 7.8 Symptoms and signs of stroke and characteristics of subtype.

Symptoms and signs of stroke

Anterior circulation strokes
- Unilateral weakness
- Unilateral sensory loss or inattention
- Isolated dysarthria
- Dysphasia
- Vision:
  Homonymous hemianopia
  Monocular blindness
  Visual inattention

Posterior circulation strokes
- Isolated homonymous hemianopia
- Diplopia and dysconjugate eyes
- Nausea and vomiting
- Incoordination and unsteadiness
- Unilateral or bilateral weakness and/or sensory loss

Nonspecific signs
- Dysphagia
- Incontinence
- Loss of consciousness

Characteristics of subtypes of stroke

	Lacunar	Partial anterior circulation	Total anterior circulation	Posterior circulation
Signs	Motor or sensory only	2 of following: motor or sensory; cortical; hemianopia	All of: motor or sensory; cortical; hemianopia	Hemianopia; brainstem; cerebellar
% dead at 1 year	10	20	60	20
% dependent at 1 year	25	30	35	20

A stroke is an acute focal neurological deficit due to a vascular lesion, lasting longer than 24 hours. A TIA is a focal neurological deficit due to a vascular lesion that resolves within 24 hours.

Onset

Obtain a chronological account of the onset and progression of neurological disability. Ask "What were you doing immediately before this happened?" Typically it occurs at rest, but patients may wake up to find that they cannot move a limb. The onset is typically immediate but may evolve over a few hours:

"One moment I was fine, the next, I was unable to move my right arm."

Define the neurological disability. For example, ask "What can't you do now that you could manage before this happened?" This is important because:
- It provides a baseline to assess recovery or subsequent deterioration.
- The anatomical site of the lesion can be identified. The neurological disability typically corresponds to the vascular territory of the occluded or hemorrhaging artery (Figs. 7.8 and 7.9).
- It allows an assessment of whether the event is likely to be a stroke or a TIA and any evidence of recovery between the onset and presentation.

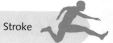

Past medical history

Consider the possible etiology of the stroke as this will affect subsequent management (Fig. 7.10). Ask specifically about previous TIAs and transient loss of sight.

Drug history

Ask specifically about warfarin, aspirin, and heparin if an intracranial bleed is suspected. Reviewing the list of medications may highlight a risk factor that the patient or his or her relatives may have forgotten.

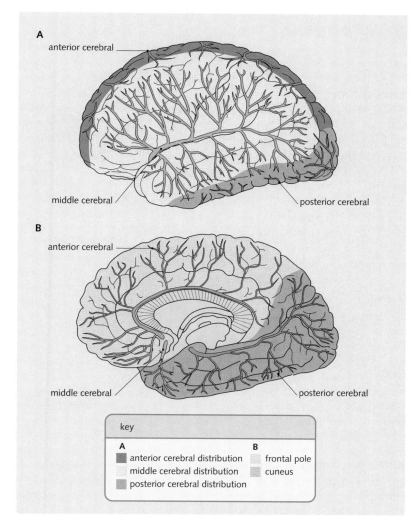

Fig. 7.9 The vascular territories of the main cerebral arteries.

Common causes of stroke	
Pathology	Features in the history
ischemic stroke*—thrombosis*, embolism*	by far the most common; ischemic heart disease, diabetes mellitus, hypertension, smoking, valvular heart disease (especially mitral stenosis/prosthetic heart valve), atrial fibrillation, family history, older age; hyperviscosity (e.g., polycythemia, Waldenström's macroglobulinemia)
cerebral hemorrhage*	common; as above, but hypertension is often pronounced; headache is often a prominent feature as is a disturbed level of consciousness
extradural hematoma	severe head injury
subdural hematoma	history of head injury (often mild); alcoholic; old age
subarachnoid hemorrhage	"herald bleeds," sudden-onset headache; loss of consciousness common; meningism
vasculitis	giant cell arteritis, systemic lupus erythematosus (SLE), Wegener's granulomatosis, sarcoidosis, etc. (consider features of above diseases)
infections	syphilis, infective endocarditis (rare)

Fig. 7.10 Etiology of strokes. Asterisks indicate the more common causes.

Social history

An extremely detailed social assessment is necessary to ascertain if and when the patient can be discharged home. Remember that discharge planning should begin at the point of admission to hospital.

The diagnosis of stroke is usually apparent on presentation, but an attempt should be made to define its etiology and severity. A large part of treatment will be supportive to aid rehabilitation. This relies upon an adequate initial assessment, and the detailed social history is essential for coordinating the various members of the multidisciplinary team (e.g., physiotherapist, occupational therapist, social worker, dietician, speech therapist).

When stroke is diagnosed, coordinate all members of the multidisciplinary team as soon as possible. Discharge planning should begin on admission to hospital.

Overview

The pediatric patient is not just a small version of an adult patient. The newborn, toddler, and adolescent have unique aspects to their histories. Clearly, a uniform approach to clinical evaluation is not applicable. Factors in the prenatal course are important, as are issues of growth and development. The HEADS mnemonic is useful when interviewing an adolescent (see below). Finally, the clinician must integrate the caregiver when the child's ability to answer questions is limited.

It is useful to distinguish the following age groups:
- Fetus: in utero.
- Neonate: birth to 28 days.
- Infant: birth to 1 year.
- Toddler: 1–3 years.
- Preschool: 3–5 years.
- School child: 5–16 years.
- Adolescent: 12–18 years.

A clinical approach for three important categories of pediatric patients is set out here:
- The adolescent.
- The toddler and preschool child aged 1–5 years.
- The infant.

Taking a history

For the majority of pediatric patients the history is taken mainly from a parent, usually the mother. The general format is the same as that in adult medicine, but with some very important differences in emphasis. Set out below is a scheme for pediatric history taking. During the history taking:
- Remember that parents, especially mothers, observe their children very closely.
- Never ignore or dismiss parental observations.
- Listen carefully: the diagnosis and the parent's concerns are usually apparent in the history.
- Avoid leading questions.

On taking a history be comprehensive: if you don't ask, they won't tell. Formulate a differential diagnosis by the end of the history. Examine the patient with your diagnosis in mind.

Introductions

On meeting the patient:
- Introduce yourself and get down to the same level as the patient (this makes you less intimidating).
- Identify the patient (find out name, age, and sex in advance). For example, "Is this Billy? How old is he?"
- Confirm the relationship of the accompanying adult. For example, "Are you his mother?" (the person could be the aunt, older sister, other relative, social worker).

Presenting complaint

Give a prompt to allow the parent to have their say, e.g., "What has been your main worry?"

Listen carefully and patiently and then follow up with specific questions to elicit the full details of presenting symptoms. The remaining parts of the pediatric medical interview differ from the adult interview in the following ways. The interview with an adolescent patient will be aided by following the suggestions at the end of this chapter.

Past medical history
Antenatal

Determine health of the mother during pregnancy. Include exposure to radiation, drugs, and infection. Include mother's previous pregnancy history.

Natal
- Duration of pregnancy.
- Birthweight.
- Kind and duration of labor.
- Type of delivery and presentation.
- Sedation and anesthesia (if known).
- State of infant at birth.
- Resuscitation required.
- Onset of respiration.
- First cry.

Neonatal

Ascertain condition of baby after birth. Determine if problems were present, such as cyanosis, jaundice, convulsions, feeding difficulties. A question about the baby's length of stay in the nursery (or if the baby went home with mother) can provide much information. Determine the need for special care, such as an incubator, transfusions, medications, and bili lights.

Growth and development
Motor and mental development
In small children, it is important to ascertain both motor and verbal milestones. When did the child first raise his/her head, roll over, sit alone, pull up, walk with help, walk alone, and talk (meaningful words; sentences) (Fig. 8.1). The Denver Developmental Screening Test (DDST) should be performed when appropriate.

In older children, school grades and quality of work are good indicators of development.

Physical growth
Gather any available data about sequential weights and lengths for later plotting on growth charts. In a young child, this would also include head circumference measurements. Any changes in usual growth pattern should be noted.

Compare the child's general growth and development with that of siblings and parents.

Nutrition
Determine the general status of the child's appetite. For infants and toddlers:
- Breast or formula: type, duration, major formula changes, time of weaning, difficulties. Be specific about how much milk or formula the baby receives.
- Vitamin supplements: type, when started, amount, duration.
- "Solid" foods: when introduced, how taken, types.

For older children:
- Obtain sample breakfast, lunch, and supper menus.

In any child with feeding difficulties or a nutritional problem, more detailed information should be obtained, such as amount taken per feeding, intervals between feedings, and presence of vomiting, crying, and weight change.

Developmental milestones				
Age	Gross motor	Fine motor and vision	Hearing and speech	Social behavior
Newborn	Symmetrical movements in all four limbs, normal muscle tone	Fixes on mother's face	Cries	Settles on being picked up
6 weeks	Good head control, presence of the Moro reflex, transiently holds head in horizontal plane when held in ventral position	Follows mother's face	Loud noises will startle them, makes contented noises	Has started to smile
8 months	Sits unsupported, starting to crawl	Palmar grasp, moves objects from hand to hand, eyes follow a dropped toy	"Dada" and "Mama," reacts to name, positive distraction test	Stranger anxiety, separation anxiety, plays "peek-a-boo"
18 months	Walks, climbs onto chair	Pincer grip, builds 3-brick tower	Three-word sentence, comprehends simple commands	Begins toilet training, uses spoon
3 years	Runs and jumps, manages stairs, kicks a ball	Builds 8-brick tower, copies lines and circles	Short sentences	Dry by day, plays with other children, dresses under supervision
5 years	Heel-toe walking, catches ball	Draws man with features	Comprehensive language skills	Can play games, tells time

Fig. 8.1 Developmental milestones.

Past illnesses

A comment should first be made relative to the child's previous general health. The specific areas listed below should then be explored:

- Infections: age, types, number, severity.
- Contagious diseases: age, complications of measles, rubella, chickenpox, mumps, pertussis, diphtheria, scarlet fever, others.
- Past hospitalizations, including operations, age, reasons for operations, complications.
- Accidents and injuries (include ingestions): nature, severity, sequelae.
- Allergies: must detail types of reaction (food, drugs, environmental agents).
- Medications that the patient is currently taking: include dosages and frequency of administration.
- Immunizations and skin tests: be familiar with departmental recommendations for immunizations. List date and type of immunization and skin tests as well as any complications or reactions. Guidelines continue to change; check a reference for current recommendations (see Appendix, p. 231).

Behavioral history

The informant should supply information as to whether the child is well adjusted or difficult to manage.

- The child's response to family members, other children, strangers, new situations, and school are clues to behavior problems.
- Does the child manifest severe and frequent temper tantrums, sleep disturbances, phobias, or pica (ingestion of substances other than food)?
- Habits: thumb sucking, nail biting, masturbation.
- Determine if there are problems with bowel and bladder training.
- For older children out of diapers, determine age at which the child was trained, presence of enuresis (lack of bladder control, day or night) and encopresis (soiling).

Special concerns for adolescents

The interview with an adolescent is a challenge! Although most of the interview is similar to the adult interview, a helpful mnemonic is HEADS (Fig. 8.2):

	Bad	Good	Reason why
Home	Tell me about mom and dad	Where do you live and who lives there with you?	Parent(s) may have died or left home. An open-ended question enables one to collect "environmental" as well as personal history.
Education	How are you doing in school?	What are you good at in school? What is hard for you? What grades do you get?	Poor questions can be "okay." Good questions ask for information about strengths and weaknesses and allow quantification.
Activities	Do you have any activities outside of school?	What do you do for fun? What things do you do with your friends? What do you do with free time?	Good questions are open-ended and allow patients to express themselves.
Drugs	Do you do drugs?	Many young people experiment with drugs, alcohol, or cigarettes. Have you or your friends ever tried them?	A good question is an expression of concern with follow-up. With younger teenagers it is best to begin by asking about friends.
Sexuality	Have you ever had sex? Tell me about your boy/girlfriend.	Have you ever had a sexual relationship with anyone? Most people become interested in sexual relationships at your age. Have you had any with boys, girls, or both? Tell me about your sex life.	What does the term "have sex" really mean to teenagers? Asking only about heterosexual relationships closes doors at once.

Examples of opening lines, good and bad

Fig. 8.2 Examples of opening lines, good and bad, for taking the history of adolescent patients.

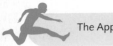

H = Home
E = Education and employment
A = Activities
D = Drugs
S = Sexuality

Review of systems

This is a set of questions used to identify key symptoms; it is similar to the adult system, with the emphasis on the system implicated by the presenting complaint:

- Respiratory system: breathing difficulties. Does the patient have any difficulty breathing while feeding?
- Cardiovascular system: syncope, breathlessness, or cyanotic episodes.
- Gastrointestinal system: appetite, vomiting, bowel habit, abdominal pain, frank weight loss, or crossing percentiles.
- Genitourinary tract: excessive thirst, polyuria, or dysuria.
- Central nervous system: headache, regression (loss of skills), or seizures.

Examination of the child

The key word in a pediatric examination is opportunistic. While in an adult examination you can have a system to work through, in pediatrics you must be flexible enough to examine what you can in the circumstances. Young infants and school-age children are relatively easy to examine, but the most commonly encountered patient in general pediatric practice is an uncooperative toddler in the 1–3-year age group. In this group particularly, the following "dos" and "don'ts" apply.

Do:

- Be friendly and cheerful. Try to smile and keep up some idle chatter (unless, of course, the child is acutely and severely ill).
- Be gentle. Rapport is lost if you cause pain or discomfort.
- Be opportunistic. If the patient is asleep, auscultate the chest; if the patient is screaming, inspect the tonsils.
- Explain or demonstrate what you are about to do; auscultate a doll or teddy bear.
- If appropriate or feasible, try and distract the child during the examination. For example, shine a pen light while examining the lung fields.

- Leave unpleasant procedures until last: examination of ears, nose, and throat, rectal examination (rarely necessary), blood pressure measurement.

Don't:

- Tower over the child.
- Stare at the child. Avoid looking too intently at toddlers.
- Separate the child from the mother. A toddler is best examined sitting on the mother's lap.
- Undress the child. Ask the mother to take off outer layers while the history is taken, but don't strip the child naked. A certain way to make toddlers cry is to undress them and lie them on a cold exam table.

The features unique to a pediatric examination of a 9-month to 5-year-old child are outlined below; the framework of "inspection, palpation, percussion, and ascultation" still holds true. For a detailed description of examination, please see the specific system chapter. The following should be read in conjunction with the specific system chapter.

General inspection

Careful initial observation should be made to assess:

- Severity of illness. Is this child well, unwell, or ill?
- Growth. Is the child well grown and well nourished? Height, weight, and head circumference should be entered on the percentile chart.
- Appearance. Are there any dysmorphic features? Is the child clean and well clothed?
- Fever or rash: infection?
- Major signs relating to specific systems: level of consciousness, pallor or bruising, cyanosis, tachypnea, or jaundice.

Hands/neck/pulse

The first touch on the hands should be gentle and nonthreatening, as should be palpation of the neck for cervical lymphadenopathy. The radial or brachial pulse can be palpated for rate, rhythm, and volume.

Chest

This includes examination of the cardiovascular and respiratory systems. Important signs common to both will have been noted on initial inspection:

- Cyanosis.
- Tachypnea (Fig. 8.3).

Pediatric vital signs			
Age	Respiratory rate	Heart rate	Systolic BP
<1	30–40	110–160	70–90
1–2	25–35	100–150	80–95
2–5	25–30	95–140	80–100
5–12	20–25	80–120	90–110
>12	15–20	60–100	100–120

Fig. 8.3 Pediatric vital signs.

- Clubbing (rare).
  In examining the respiratory system, look for:
- Intercostal or subcostal retraction.
- Nasal flaring.
- Use of accessory muscles.
- Chest shape and movement specifically, including asymmetrical movements.

Percuss (but this is seldom helpful in very young infants).
Auscultate and note:
- Breath sounds.
- Added sounds (e.g., wheeze and crackles).

The cardiovascular system should be examined as described in Chapter 4. Detailed evaluation includes:
- Measuring blood pressure (this is quite unpleasant for a child and so should be left until the end if possible).
- Checking for hepatomegaly: this is an important sign of cardiac failure in infants.

Additional features in the examination of the abdomen
Inspect for:
- Distension, which may be due to intestinal obstruction or ascites.
- Peristalsis, which is a useful sign in pyloric stenosis.
- Inguinal region and genitalia (hernia, hydrocele, testicular torsion).

Palpate the abdomen for tenderness or guarding.

Masses/organomegaly
Auscultate and listen to the bowel sounds, which are:
- Increased in obstruction and acute diarrhea.
- Reduced in ileus.
- Absent in peritonitis.

Rectal examination may be indicated in suspected appendicitis or intussusception. Remember that this is an unpleasant procedure. Try to have a parent in the room with you for reassurance and use your little finger.

Nervous system
Important signs noted on inspection include:
- Level of consciousness.
- Which developmental milestones have been met (as in Fig. 8.1).

In infants, it is important to:
- Measure occipitofrontal head circumference.
- Palpate the anterior fontanelle: this is a window in the skull that allows assessment of intracranial pressure and levels of dehydration. It closes at about 12 months.

If indicated, more detailed evaluation may include the same features as would be examined in an adult: tone, power, coordination, sensation, and reflexes (see Chapter 18).

Ears and throat
Usually left to the last, as their examination is not enjoyed by toddlers, mothers, or doctors. The key to success is parental help in holding the child. The child should be seated on the mother's lap and held firmly by her with one hand on the forehead and one around the trunk and both arms.
Examine the ears first and the throat last; the occasional child will cooperate by "opening wide." In some cases it is necessary to insert a wooden spatula between clenched teeth onto the tongue.

Examination of the infant

Routine examination
As soon as a baby is born, the obstetrician, family physician (or pediatrician if present) will check that the baby is pink, breathing normally, and has no major congenital malformations. Obviously, if the infant is of low birthweight (<2500 g) or ill (e.g., after-birth asphyxia), admission to a special care baby unit will be required.
About 95% of babies are born at term and appear healthy. However, they all need a full medical

examination within the first 24 hours of life. The purpose of this is:
- To give the parents a chance to ask any questions about their baby.
- To identify any problems anticipated as a result of maternal disease or familial disorders (e.g., congenital infection, maternal diabetes mellitus).
- To detect congenital abnormalities, which may not be immediately obvious at birth (e.g., cataract, cleft palate, heart murmur, undescended testes, dislocatable hip).

A scheme for the routine examination of the normal term infant is outlined below.

Look hard but unobtrusively before you touch. Careful observation is the key to success.

Vital information is obtained just from looking.

Upper airways noises are readily transmitted to the upper chest in infants. They can be difficult to distinguish from coarse rhonchi.

Watch a child's face for grimaces as you palpate the abdomen.

Putting the child's hand under yours may enhance cooperation.

In the first 24 hours, many babies have a quiet systolic "flow" murmur. Features suggesting a significant murmur:
- Loud murmur.
- Diastolic murmur.
- Associated cardiac signs.

- These should be investigated with chest x-ray, ECG, and echocardiogram.

To test for congenital dislocation of the hip, use the:
- Barlow manuever: stabilize the pelvis with one hand and with the other abduct the hip to 45°. If the hip is dislocated, forward pressure with your middle finger will cause the femoral head to slip back into the acetabulum.
- Ortolani maneuver: with the child on his/her back, flex the hips to 90° and also bend the knees to 90°. Place your middle finger over the greater trochanter and your thumb on the inner aspect of the thigh over the lesser trochanter. The child has a dislocated hip if slow abduction causes a palpable or audible jolt. A click is more commonly felt and is not diagnostic of a dislocated hip.

After the child has been discharged from hospital, he or she should have multiple visits with the primary care physician. These will include:
- Weight and head circumference.
- Hips again.
- Testes and penis.
- Heart sounds.
- Primitive reflexes.
- Muscle tone.
- Smiling.
- And most importantly, any parental concerns?

9. Presenting Problems in Psychiatric Patients

Overview

Psychiatry can be a challenging area of medicine. It also makes up more of the workload than you may at first imagine. Around a quarter of the population may experience some form of psychiatric symptom in a year. At any given time roughly 7% of the population will have depression, and the lifetime risk of schizophrenia is 1% (remember that schizophrenia carries a 10% lifetime risk of suicide). Patients with physical disease may also (and often do) develop mental distress as part of their reaction to ill health.

Psychiatric disease presents with disorders of mood, thoughts, or behavior. Psychiatric disease can be categorized into four areas:

- Brain diseases, including dementia, delirium, schizophrenia, and bipolar disorder.
- Personality traits with psychiatric significance, such as mental retardation, unstable introversion, or extroversion.
- Behavior disorders, including alcoholism, drug addiction, eating disorders, and hysteria.
- Disorders related to life events such as grief, depression, and situational anxiety.

Tests of cognitive function such as the mini-mental status exam and the more detailed mental status exam are critically important in the patient presenting with psychiatric disease.

With psychiatric problems, more so than any other area, history taking is key. It can be very difficult as patients may be too distressed or unwilling to communicate. Developing a rapport is essential but can be very challenging.

Remember your safety. It may be advisable to have a chaperone with you, but this is not always possible or appropriate. Always make sure that the patient does not come between you and the door.

The following is an outline of the format of a psychiatric history and the mental state examination.

A thumbnail sketch

This should include the patient's name, age, and occupation.

Presenting complaint

Always ask open questions: "What brought you to see a psychiatrist?" or "Why do you think you're here?" As with all histories, it is important to use the words that the patient used (e.g., "Life just isn't worth living").

History of the presenting complaint

As discussed in Chapter 2, it is important to formulate an idea of how long this has been going on. Is it gradual in onset, or is it acute? Have there been any clear precipitants (e.g., drug-induced psychosis)? Does anything make this better, does anything make it worse? How often does this happen? Is it weekly, daily, or even monthly? It is important to get an idea of how severe an impact on the patient's life the problem is having. Ask if it is interfering with employment and relationships.

Past psychiatric history

Has this person had contact with psychiatric services previously? For example, have there been depressive episodes or deliberate self-harm? What was the form of this? Have they been admitted to hospital, and have they ever had psychotherapy or counseling? Each episode should be investigated and detailed. Many psychiatric disorders are chronic and so there has often been multiple contacts with the patient. You might also ask about ongoing contact with psychiatric services, community mental health teams, partial hospitalization, and/or regular visits to a primary care physician).

Family history

This is generally split into two sections.

Relationships with parents and siblings

Do they get along with their family, and what contact do they have with them? Is home a safe and supportive place to be? What have been the learned coping mechanisms that they have developed? For example, you might ask, "In the past when you felt down, what actions have you taken?" Do any family members have criminal convictions. If so, for what? The answer might be "Dad has spent the last 10 years in prison."

Family psychiatric history

Since many psychiatric illnesses have a genetic component, it is important to know if any family members have psychiatric illnesses.

Personal history
Early development

Were there any problems during pregnancy or at birth? Did the patient meet developmental milestones? (See Chapter 8.) If the patient is young enough, you may have access to one or both parents to ask these questions; otherwise you will have to ask patients if they can recall either parent discussing their early childhood.

Childhood behavior

Did they play with other children, or were they antisocial? You will need to explore the possibility that the person may have been abused at some point in childhood. This is a difficult area to broach, and not everyone will volunteer the information at the first time of asking. A more oblique approach may be helpful. For example, you can make a statement (e.g., "Sometimes distressing experiences in childhood can make people feel this way") instead of asking a question.

School history

What kind of school did they attend? For example, was it a single-sex, boarding, or juvenile correctional institution? Were they bullied, or did they do the bullying? Did they manage to make and maintain friendships at school? Were they often absent? What was their disciplinary record like (e.g., suspensions and expulsions)? Were there any family upheavals during these years (e.g., divorce, deaths in the family)?

Occupational history

Ask how many jobs they have had, how long they kept the jobs, and why they left (e.g., the 16-year-old boy who went into mining and was then fired and has not found work in the past 10 years).

Sexual history

This includes sexual orientation, number of partners (including use of prostitutes), and whether or not relationships have been successful.

Relationship/marriage

Often this is quite different from the above. Has the person been in a stable relationship that has recently ended and so they have lost their social support network?

Children

How many children do they have and with how many partners? What sort of contact do they have with the children, and how do they feel about this?

Forensic history

Have they ever been in trouble with the police? If so, how much contact was there? Have they been to prison? If so, for how long and how many times? Do they have a case pending?

Current social circumstances

With whom are they living at present? Where are they living? Are they the owner-occupier, or is it a rented accommodation? How many people live there? The answers to these questions can be quite revealing.

Premorbid personality

It is important to ask patients how they perceived themselves before they became ill. Ask them about the following topics.

Social relationships

Do they feel that they get along with people? Did they have a social support network? Who were their friends, and how did they perceive the relationships?

Hobbies/interests

For example, find out if patients like sports or have a hobby like model railways. Are they members of any clubs?

Predominant mood

Would they describe themselves as predominantly anxious, pessimistic, depressed, happy, or optimistic? The number of people who describe themselves as happy-go-lucky is amazing!

Character

Would they describe themselves generally as irritable, self-centered, obsessive, or suspicious?

History of risk-taking behaviors

Do they drink alcohol? If so, how much? Do they use recreational drugs? If so, which drugs do they use (e.g., amphetamines, ecstasy, cannabis, heroin, tobacco)? It is important to quantify drug use. A full and comprehensive drug history is essential.

Past medical history

This is no different from taking a history in any other setting, but remember particularly to ask about previous head injuries and epilepsy. Medical problems can have psychological presentations or sequelae (e.g., hypothyroidism). Ask about medications, which also may cause psychiatric problems.

A full psychiatric history can take upward of an hour. Do not worry if the patient chooses to terminate the interview. Very often more than one interview is required to build rapport and thus obtain a full picture.

The mental state examination

This is the psychiatrist's equivalent of the physical examination. It begins when you first meet the patient and continues throughout the interview. It is your assessment of the patient's mental state at the time you see him/her and not the history of the patient's illness. In the routine medical interview, Folstein's Mini Mental Exam (Fig. 9.1) can be performed. The complete mental status exam is demonstrated below and is broken into the following parts:

Observed during interview

- Appearance
- Behavior
- Level of consciousness

- Emotional state
- Speech
- Form of thought
- Perceptual symptoms
- Thought content and complex systems

Tested functions

- Gross motor function
- Orientation
- Attention and concentration
- Memory
- Information
- Vocabulary
- Abstract thinking
- Judgment and comprehension

Data collected

Observed during interview

Appearance

- The patient is a ____ Black, ____ White, ____ Hispanic, ____ Asian, ____ Indian, ____ male, ____ female in ____ no, ____ moderate, ____ severe distress.
- He or she is ____ obese, ____ well nourished, ____ emaciated and appears ____ older than, ____ younger than, ____ the stated age.
- The patient's dress and grooming appear ____ neat, ____ disheveled, ____ casual, ____ formal, ____ clean, ____ dirty, ____ attention-seeking, ____ immature, ____ seductive, ____ bizarre (describe)_____.
- The patient's hair is ____ neatly groomed, ____ clean, ____ dirty, ____ filthy, with ____ no ____ noticeable, ____ intense body odor.

Behavior

- The patient appears ____ relaxed, ____ agitated, ____ hyperactive, ____ hypoactive, and has ____ mannerisms (describe) _____, ____ posturing (describe)_____, ____ rigidity.
- The patient relates to the examiner in a ____ pleasant, ____ cooperative, ____ hostile, ____ uncooperative, ____ guarded, ____ apprehensive, ____ bewildered, ____ seductive, ____ threatening, ____ assaultive, ____ manipulative, ____ trusting, ____ dependent, ____ suspicious way, ____ indifferently.

Level of consciousness

- The patient appears to be ____ comatose, ____ stuporous, ____ lethargic, ____ alert, ____ hypervigilant.

73

FOLSTEIN MINI-MENTAL STATUS EXAM

Patient Score	Maximum Score	

Orientation

_____ 5   What is the (year) (season) (date) (day) (month)?

_____ 5   Where are we (country) (state) (county) (city) (clinic)?

Registration

_____ 3   Name three objects, allotting one second to say each one. Then ask the patient to name all three objects after you have said them. Give one point for each correct answer. Repeat them until patient hears all three. Count trials and record number

APPLE...BOOK...COAT   Number of trials _____

Attention and Calculation

_____ 5   Begin with 100 and count backward by 7 (stop after five answers): 93, 86, 79, 72, 65. Score one point for each correct answer. If the patient will not perform this task, ask the patient to spell WORLD backwards (DLROW). Record the patient's spelling: _____ Score one point for each correctly placed letter.

Recall

_____ 3   Ask the patient to repeat the objects above (see Registration). Give one point for each correct answer.

Language

_____ 2   Naming: Show a pencil and a watch, and ask the patient to name them.
_____ 1   Repetition: Repeat the following: "No ifs, ands, or buts."
_____ 3   Three-stage command: Follow the three-stage command, "Take a paper in your right hand; fold it in half; and put it on the table."
_____ 1   Reading: Read and obey the following: "Close your eyes."
_____ 1   Writing: Write a sentence.
_____ 1   Copying: Copy the design of the intersecting pentagons.

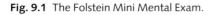

_____ 30   **Total Score**

Adapted from Folstein MF, Folstein S, McHugh PR. Mini-mental state: A practical method for grading the cognitive state of patients for the clinician. *J Psychiatr Res* 1975;12:189-198.

Fig. 9.1 The Folstein Mini Mental Exam.

Emotional state

- The patient's predominant affective response is
  ____ sadness, ____ joy, ____ fear, ____ anger,
  ____ unremarkable. Range of affect is ____ flat,
  ____ constricted, ____ varied. Affect is
  ____ appropriate, ____ inappropriate to the
  situation and to thought content.
- The patient's mood is ____ depressed,
  ____ euphoric, ____ apathetic, ____ optimistic,
  ____ pessimistic, ____ unremarkable.

You must ask directly about suicidal ideation at some point. Failure to do so will be considered negligent.

Speech

- The patient speaks ____ slowly, ____ rapidly,
  ____ at normal rate.
- Latency of response is ____ long, ____ short,
  ____ unremarkable. Voice quality is ____ loud,
  ____ soft, ____ normal, ____ variable in pitch,
  ____ high-pitched, ____ low-pitched,
  ____ monotonal. Speech is ____ pressured,
  ____ not pressured.

Form of thought

- The patient's form of thought is ____
  unremarkable, ____ remarkable as evidenced by
  ____ loose associations, ____ tangential thinking,
  ____ circumstantiality, ____ neologisms,
  ____ perserveration, ____ thought blocking,
  ____ clang associations. The patient appears
  ____ aphasic, ____ not aphasic. The aphasia
  appears to be ____ fluent, ____ nonfluent.

Perceptual symptoms

- The patient demonstrates evidence of
  hallucinations by appearing to ____ look at,
  ____ feel, ____ smell, ____ hear, ____ taste
  something not perceived by the examiner.
- The patient demonstrates evidence of illusions by
  misinterpeting a ____ sound, ____ sight,
  ____ smell, ____ taste, or ____ touch.

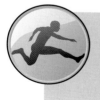

Visual hallucinations point toward an organic problem, whereas auditory hallucinations are commonly associated with schizophrenia.

Thought content and complex symptoms

- The patient expresses ____ no delusions.
  Delusions that are ____ grandiose,
  ____ persecutory, ____ somatic, ____ of poverty
  or guilt, of control, influence of reference
  (underline which). The patient demonstrates
  ____ thought broadcasting, ____ obsessions
  (describe) _____, ____ compulsions
  (describe) _____, ____ phobias (describe)
  _____, ____ free-floating anxiety,
  ____ depersonalization or derealization
  (underline), ____ déjà vu or similar experience.

Tested functions

Gross motor function

- The patient appears ____ coordinated,
  ____ uncoordinated, and ____ can ____ cannot
  manipulate objects and do simple manual tasks.

Orientation

- The patient is ____ oriented, ____ disoriented to
  ____ day, ____ month, ____ year.
- If disoriented to above, is also disoriented to
  ____ time of day, ____ season.
- Patient is disoriented to the ____ location,
  ____ type of place, ____ city, ____ state,
  ____ country. The patient is ____ oriented,
  ____ disoriented to his own person (describe)
  _____.

Attention and concentration

Digit span

Digits forward	Digits backward
3, 8, 6	2, 5
6, 1, 2	6, 3
3, 4, 1, 7	5, 7, 4
6, 1, 5, 8	2, 5, 9
8, 4, 2, 3, 9	7, 2, 9, 6
5, 2, 1, 8, 6	8, 4, 1, 3
3, 8, 9, 1, 7, 4	4, 1, 6, 2, 7
7, 9, 6, 4, 8, 3	9, 7, 8, 5, 2
5, 1, 7, 4, 2, 3, 8	1, 6, 5, 2, 9, 8
9, 8, 5, 2, 1, 6, 3	3, 6, 7, 2, 9, 4
1, 6, 4, 5, 9, 7, 6, 3	8, 5, 9, 2, 3, 4, 2
2, 9, 7, 6, 3, 1, 5, 4	4, 5, 7, 9, 2, 8, 1
5, 3, 8, 7, 1, 2, 4, 6, 9	6, 9, 1, 6, 3, 2, 5, 8
4, 2, 6, 9, 1, 7, 8, 3, 5	3, 1, 7, 9, 5, 4, 8, 2

Serial 7s The patient was able to do serial 7s
____ with no mistakes, ____ with 3 or fewer mistakes,
____ with more than 3 mistakes, ____ with a few
mistakes, ____ poorly. Record answers and time.

Memory

Recent memory   The patient's recent memory is
____ intact, ____ impaired as evidenced by,
____ cannot recall three objects in a few minutes,
____ cannot recall hospital staff names, procedures,
events known to examiner.

Remote memory   The patient cannot recall
____ president, ____ president before him, ____ vice
president, ____ governor, ____ mayor, ____ date of
birth, ____ date of anniversary.

Information

1. How many days are there in a week?
2. What must you do to water to make it boil?
3. How many things are in a dozen?
4. Name the four seasons of the year.
5. What do we celebrate on the 4th of July?
6. How many pounds are there in a ton?
7. What does the stomach do?
8. What is the capital of Greece?
9. Where does the sun set?
10. Who invented the airplane?
11. Why does oil float on water?
12. Where do we get turpentine from?
13. When is Labor Day?
14. How far is it from New York to Chicago?
15. What is a hieroglyphic?
16. What is a barometer?
17. Who wrote *Paradise Lost*?
18. What is a prime number?
19. What is Habeas Corpus?
20. Who discovered the South Pole?

Vocabulary (record what patient says)

1. Apple
2. Donkey
3. Diamond
4. Nuisance
5. Join
6. Fur
7. Dime
8. Bacon
9. Tint
10. Armory
11. Fable
12. Nitroglycerin
13. Microscope
14. Stanza
15. Guillotine
16. Plural
17. Seclude
18. Spangle
19. Recede
20. Affliction
21. Chattel
22. Dilatory
23. Flout
24. Amanuensis

Abstract thinking (record patient's interpretation verbatim; discontinue after 4 consecutive failures)

1. Proverbs:
   - Don't count your chickens before they are hatched.
   - There is no use crying over spilled milk.
   - The wheel that does the squeaking gets the grease.
   - A stitch in times saves nine.
   - As the twig is bent, so is the tree inclined.
   - You can catch more flies with honey than vinegar.
   - It's an ill wind that blows nobody good.
   - The restless sleeper blames the couch.
   - The tongue is the enemy of the neck.
   - The mouse that has but one hole is soon caught.
2. Similarities:
   - A plum and a peach
   - Beer and wine
   - Cat and mouse
   - Piano and violin
   - Paper and coal
   - Pound and yard
   - Scissors and copper pan
   - Mountain and lake
   - First and last
   - Salt and water
   - Liberty and justice
   - Forty-nine and one hundred and twenty-one

Judgment and comprehension

1. What is the thing to do if you lose a book belonging to a library?
2. Why is it better to build a house with brick than with wood?
3. What should you do if you see a train approaching a broken track?
4. Why is it generally better to give money to an organized charity than to a street beggar?
5. What is the thing to do if a very good friend asks you for something that you don't have?
6. Why are criminals locked up or put in prison?

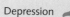

7. Why should most government positions be filled through Civil Service Examinations?
8. Why does the United States require that a person wait at least two years from the time he makes application until the time he receives his final citizen papers?
9. Why is cotton used in making cloth?
10. Why should a promise be kept?

Depression

Depression as an isolated symptom is one of the commonest presenting complaints that primary care physicians see. It often presents in both hospital and community settings with vague physical symptoms (e.g., tiredness). It is easily missed, and accurate diagnosis depends upon the communication skills of the doctor. When taking a history from a depressed patient, open and closed questions are needed. It is important to elucidate any of the symptoms listed in Fig. 9.2 and must include suicidal intent. It is a myth that asking a patient about suicidal ideation will precipitate the thought in their minds. It is negligent to fail to ascertain any such ideation. It is often possible to ask a direct question (e.g., "Have you ever been so unhappy that you've thought about ending

Characteristics of major depression: SIGECAPS interview

- Sleep disorder (either increased or decreased sleep)*
- Interests deficit (anhedonia)
- Guilt (worthlessness,* hopelessness,* regret)
- Energy deficit*
- Concentration deficit*
- Appetite (either decreased or increased)*
- Psychomotor agitation or slowing
- Suicidal ideation

Fig. 9.2 Characteristics of major depression: SIGECAPS interview. To meet the diagnosis of major depression, a patient must have four of the symptoms plus depressed mood or anhedonia, for at least two weeks. To meet the diagnosis of dysthymic disorder, a patient must have two of the six symptoms marked with an asterisk, plus depression, for at least two years.

your life?"), but it may be more appropriate to ask in a more oblique fashion (e.g., "Sometimes when people are so unhappy, they feel that they can't go on?"). It is important to differentiate between real suicidal intent and the more common feeling that a patient wishes that he or she were dead but has no intention of taking his/her own life. This may require direct but sensitive probing.

10. Presenting Problems: Musculoskeletal System

Overview

Patients with disorders of the musculoskeletal system often have rheumatic disease. These patients present with joint pain or inflammation of many organs. Patients with multisystem disease challenge the clinician to find clues from many sources, including the eyelids, nailbeds, and constitutional symptoms of fatigue.

When approaching the patient with joint pain, we need to ascertain the presence or absence of inflammation, the number of joints involved, and the sites and distribution of the involved joints. Important clues include the pattern of joint pain, the presence of extra-articular symptoms, the age and sex of the patient, and the family history.

Back pain

History of present illness

Back pain is extremely common. It is the largest single cause of lost working hours in the developed world among both manual and sedentary workers; in the former it is an important cause of long-term disability. The history is used to highlight potentially serious or treatable causes of the pain. Consider the differential diagnosis of back pain (Fig. 10.1).

Ask patients what they think is causing the pain. This is always extremely informative. Take a detailed history in the usual systematic manner, focusing on the factors below.

Location/radiation

Most back pain is in the lumbar region. Thoracic pain is usually due to an organic cause (e.g., tuberculosis, osteoporotic compression fracture, myeloma). Back pain often radiates to other sites; for example, radiation down the distribution of the sciatic nerve after lumbar disk prolapse.

Onset

Onset may be acute (e.g., disk prolapse, compression fracture), insidious (e.g., malignancy, infection, inflammatory causes), or chronic for years (nonspecific back pain).

Modifying factors

Mechanical pain is often exacerbated by exercise. Inflammatory pain is often worse after a period of inactivity. Spinal stenosis may be worse on walking but relieved by leaning forward or resting.

Pattern of severity with time

For example, is the patient experiencing chronic unrelenting pain (e.g., inflammatory disease, psychogenic), intermittent, or relapsing pain (e.g., disk disease)?

Associated symptoms

A full review of systems should be performed bcause the back pain may be part of a systemic disease such as ankylosing spondylosis (e.g., polyarthritis, dyspnea), malignancy, renal failure (e.g., hypercalcemia).

Past medical history

A detailed past medical history may elicit a potential underlying cause for the pain. Consider psychiatric disorders, especially depression, which may be a cause or result of the pain (e.g., somatization or lowered pain threshold).

Drug history

Ask patients what analgesics they have taken in an attempt to relieve the symptoms and their efficacy.

Social history

Explore how the pain limits functional activity. Ask specifically about time off work due to the pain. For suspected nonspecific pain or psychogenic pain, explore current social pressures experienced by the patient.

Review of systems

It is essential to consider systemic illnesses that may have precipitated the pain. In particular, consider weight loss, fevers, sweats, features suggestive of malignancy, and polyarthritis.

Differential diagnosis of back pain
Inflammatory ankylosing spondylitis*; psoriatic arthropathy; enteropathic arthropathy
Bone disease osteoporosis*; osteomalacia; renal bone disease; malignancy
Disk disease and osteoarthritis spondylosis*; acute disk prolapse*; tuberculosis and septic diskitis
Mechanical disease posture* (pregnancy, obesity, scoliosis, etc.); spondylolisthesis; spinal stenosis
Soft tissue disease "fibrositis"; muscle strain* Back pain is unlikely to have a serious cause when: • the patient can get on and off the examination table without discomfort • there is no associated spasm of the spinal muscles and/or local tenderness • the spine has a full range of movement
Nonspecific back pain* the most common cause; usually has a mechanical basis
Referred pain chronic pancreatitis; posterior duodenal ulcer; abdominal aortic aneurysm, etc.

Fig. 10.1 Differential diagnosis of back pain. Asterisks indicate more common causes.

 Back pain is very common. A good history is the key to efficient diagnosis and can prevent unnecessary and occasionally expensive or unpleasant investigations, which may reinforce illness behavior. Try to distinguish between systemic disease and mechanical pain. Symptoms such as thoracic pain, weight loss, fevers, systemic symptoms, or new-onset pain should trigger alarm bells. Psychogenic back pain is a diagnosis of exclusion. An attempt to make a positive diagnosis should be made so that management can be tailored to the diagnosis.

Rheumatoid arthritis

History of present illness

Rheumatoid arthritis is a multisystem disease, and the history should be taken in a systematic manner.

Background disease

Ask about age of onset (typically 25–40 years) and usual pattern of arthritis. About 5–10% of patients will have a positive family history.

Current disease activity

Attempt to assess whether the patient has active synovitis, and try to distinguish it from secondary osteoarthritis due to burnt-out rheumatoid disease. Inquire about the time pattern of disease activity (e.g., relentless progression, disease flares separated by periods of remission) and the presence of red or swollen joints. If so, note the response to analgesics and nonsteroidal anti-inflammatory drugs (NSAIDs) and the duration of early morning stiffness (>30 minutes is significant). Map out the joints that the patient thinks are inflamed (Fig. 10.2).

Functional impact of the disease

Consider how current disease activity has altered functional ability. For example, ask "Is there anything that you have difficulty doing now that you could manage a few weeks ago?" Consider mobility, grip, doing buttons, climbing stairs. Ascertain whether activities are limited by pain, weakness, or other factors.

Fig. 10.2 Simple diagrams can be used to illustrate the distribution of active synovitis. Shaded circles represent inflamed joints.

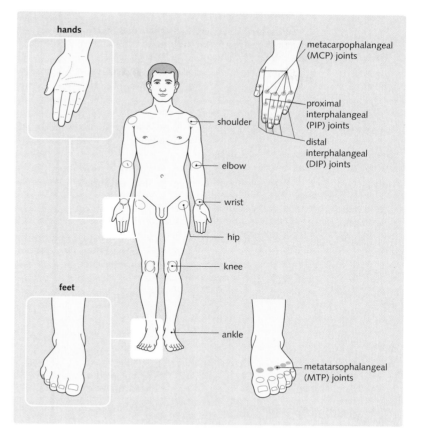

Extra-articular features of the disease

Rheumatoid arthritis should be considered as a systemic disease. For each system, consider how disease activity may be manifested:

- Lung: dyspnea (e.g., due to rheumatoid nodules, pleural effusion, bronchiolitis obliterans).
- Skin: rash, vasculitic leg ulcers, rheumatoid nodules.
- Nervous system: paresthesias (especially carpal tunnel syndrome), symptoms of peripheral neuropathy.
- Eyes: dry eyes (Sjögren's syndrome), especially if associated with a dry mouth, red eye (scleritis).
- Renal: proteinuria or known dysfunction (e.g., due to amyloid, medication).
- Anemia: many patients have an anemia of chronic disease; this may be exacerbated by anemia due to blood loss if the patient is on NSAIDs.

Drug history

A particularly detailed drug history is absolutely essential. Concentrate on drugs currently being used to control the disease (e.g., steroids, analgesics, NSAIDs, disease-modifying agents). Often a multitude of drug combinations has been used previously. Try to chart previous experiences objectively so that an assessment can be made about changing agents, if necessary, to improve control of disease activity. For each disease-modifying agent, chart:

- Acceptability of agent to the patient.
- Time period of use.
- Efficacy: use objective and subjective parameters, if possible; for example, the patient's self-report, early morning stiffness, erythrocyte sedimentation rate (ESR), progression of joint erosions radiologically.
- Reason for discontinuation (e.g., side effects, lack of response).
- Doses used, especially cumulative dose.
- If patients are taking NSAIDs, have they had any gastrointestinal side effects?

All second-line agents have side effects (Fig. 10.3). Ask specifically about the use of steroids.

Side effects of second-line agents used in the treatment of rheumatoid arthritis			
Drug	**Brand name(s)**	**Dosage**	**Side effects**
auranofin (oral gold)	Ridaura	6–9 mg per day in 1 or 2 doses	proteinuria (membranous nephropathy); thrombocytopenia and agranulocytosis; skin rash (approximately 25%); stomatitis
azathioprine	Imuran	50–150 mg per day in 1 to 3 doses	bone marrow suppression; increased risk of malignancy; infections; gastrointestinal disturbances
chlorambucil	Leukeran	2–8 mg per day in 1 or 2 doses	moderate suppression blood counts; acute leukemia in 5–10% with prolonged treatment; temporary or permanent aspermia or amenorrhea
cyclophosphamide	Cytoxan	50–150 mg per day in a single dose orally (this drug may also be given intravenously)	moderate suppression blood counts; alopecia, hemorrhagic cystitis; temporary or permanent aspermia or amenorrhea
cyclosporine	Neoral, Sandimmune	100–400 mg per day in 2 doses	nephrotoxicity, hepatotoxicity, hypertension and malignant lymphoma
gold sodium thiomalate (injectable gold)	Myochrysine	10 mg in a single injection the first week, 25 mg the following week, then 25–50 mg per week thereafter. Frequency may be reduced after several months.	proteinuria (membranous nephropathy); thrombocytopenia and agranulocytosis; skin rash (approximately 25%); stomatitis
hydroxychloroquine sulfate	Plaquenil	200–600 mg per day in 1 or 2 doses	retinopathy (especially long-term use)
leflunomide	Arava	10–20 mg per day in a single dose	diarrhea, rash, reversible alopecia, and hepatotoxicity. Occasional unexplained dramatic weight loss. Carcinogenic and teratogenic
methotrexate	Rheumatrex, Trexall	7.5–20 mg per week in a single dose orally (this drug may also be given by injection)	bone marrow suppression; oral ulceration; gastrointestinal disturbances; hepatotoxicity (especially prolonged use); teratogenic
minocycline	Minocin	200 mg per day in 2 doses	uncommon except for dizziness (10%)
penicillamine	Cuprimine, Depen	125–250 mg per day in a single dose to start, increased to not more than 1500 mg per day in 3 doses	proteinuria (common); nephritic syndrome; thrombocytopenia; agranulocytosis; anorexia; nausea (early in treatment); rash
sulfasalazine	Azulfidine, Azulfidine EN-Tabs	500–3000 mg to 3g per day in 2 to 4 doses	sulfasalazine nausea; vomiting; skin rash; blood dyscrasia (rare)

Fig. 10.3 Side effects of second-line agents used in the treatment of rheumatoid arthritis.

Social history

It is important to investigate the functional impact of the disease on daily life, exploring the home environment as well as occupation. Many aids to living are available, and specialist use of physiotherapists and occupational therapists may be invaluable. As with many long-term disabling conditions, it is easy to concentrate on symptom control and practical issues; inquire how the patient is feeling and coping and what they are worried about. This is equally important.

Remember that rheumatoid arthritis is a chronic (and often disabling) condition. Patient education and motivation are crucial for optimal rehabilitation. It is particularly important to foster an air of mutual trust between the patient and doctor.

Osteoarthritis

This is the most common joint condition and is three times more common in women than men. It normally presents at about age 50 years. It usually occurs as a primary feature but may occur after injury. Patients normally complain about pain on exertion that is relieved by rest. The pain is often worse at the end of the day. This process begins insidiously and develops over years. With time the relief with rest is less complete. The patient may also complain about stiffness after periods of rest. Unlike the inflammatory joint diseases, however, there are no systemic features of osteoarthritis.

Ask the patient which joints are particularly affected: (in order) the distal interphalangeal joints, first metacarpophalangeal joints, and first metatarsophalangeal joints are most commonly affected. The hip and knees are also commonly affected. Determine the patient's current level of function and what exactly stops him/her from doing more. It is useful to find out if patients have had any joint replacements and whether they feel that they have been successful. Because patients often complain about pain, it is important to take a drug history to determine what analgesics they use and which they find most effective. Refer to Chapter 22 on imaging for detail about the x-ray changes associated with osteoarthritis.

Perthes' disease

This condition is a subject much loved of orthopedic surgeons as it demonstrates the changing anatomy of the blood supply to the hip with age. It is a disease of childhood and has an incidence of 1 : 10 000. The patient is usually a boy between the ages of 4 and 8 with delayed skeletal maturity. (Boys are four times more affected than girls.) Initially patients complain of hip pain and then start to limp. The joint is irritable; thus, all movements are diminished and painful at the extremes. Abduction and internal rotation are the most commonly affected movements.

Between the ages of 4 and 7 the femoral head is dependent on the lateral epiphyseal vessels for its blood supply. Their course makes them susceptible to occlusion by pressure from any effusion around the hip. After the age of 7 the blood vessels in the ligamentum terres are developed and supply the femoral head.

The pathology is a three-stage process. Initially, there are one or more episodes of ischemia causing bone death. Revascularization and repair then occur, with distortion and remodeling of the femoral head and neck. This can then lead to the incomplete covering of the femoral head by the acetabulum.

Slipped capital femoral epiphysis

A slipped capital femoral epiphysis is basically a fracture through the hypertrophic zone of the cartilaginous growth plate. The patient is usually a pubertal boy who presents with referred hip pain (e.g., knee pain, groin pain, anterior thigh pain, and limping). They can present with acute pain following trauma, chronically or with acute-on-chronic pain. These patients are often overweight and sexually underdeveloped. On examination the leg will be externally rotated and shorter and all movements will be painful.

Fractured neck of femur

This fracture usually happens to older women who have osteoporosis. It often follows a simple fall; however, care should be taken to insure that there is no medical cause for the fall. The patient cannot normally bear weight, but some are able to walk, albeit with considerable pain. On examination, the affected limb is shortened and externally rotated. This condition has a 1-year mortality rate of approximately 50%. The fractures are classified according to Garden's classification (Fig. 10.4; see also Chapter 22 on imaging). Patients are often frail and susceptible to hospital-acquired pneumonia, pressure sores, DVT, and PEs. If the patient is to make a successful recovery, operative management is mandatory to facilitate early mobilization.

Garden's classification of fractured neck of femur	
Type 1	Inferior cortex not completely broken but trabecule lines are angulated
Type 2	Inferior cortex clearly broken but trabecule lines are not angulated
Type 3	Obvious fracture line and rotation of head in acetabulum
Type 4	Fully displaced fracture

Fig. 10.4 Garden's classification of fractured neck of femur.

11. Presenting Problems: Endocrine System

Overview

Disorders of the endocrine system are continually becoming more common with the obesity epidemic ravaging the U.S. Although some specific symptoms are associated with diabetes (polyuria, polydipsia, and polyphagia), many diseases of the endocrine system present with common and nonspecific symptoms. These include the weakness and fatigue in adrenal insufficiency or the weight changes in thyroid disorders. Considering functional disorders, the clinician may attribute these symptoms to stress or other illness. Thus, endocrine and metabolic disorders require physicians to maintain a high index of suspicion.

The diabetic patient

Form of diabetes mellitus

Note the class of disease, since complications and management strategies vary:
- Type 1: lack of insulin.
- Type 2: insulin resistance.
- Secondary (due to glucocorticosteroids, pancreatitis, Cushing's disease).

Diabetic control

This is the cornerstone of managing diabetes mellitus, so much of the time available at consultation should be devoted to diabetic control. Review the form of blood sugar control (e.g., diet alone, oral hypoglycemic agents, insulin). Try and ascertain adherence. Be sensitive in inquiring; for example, "Do you ever forget to take your tablets?" or "Do you have dietary lapses?"

Establish how the patient monitors glycemic control. Check the form of monitoring (e.g., measuring blood glucose), frequency of measurements, and the levels attained. Most patients have a book charting the blood glucose level. Some monitors allow downloading of blood glucose values to a computer, or you can scroll through values directly on the monitor. These values should be reviewed to assess general control and fluctuations at different times of the day. They also provide an additional insight into the patient's adherence. In an analogous way to checking inhaler technique, it is often informative to observe a patient performing a blood glucose estimate. While patients may try to improve their diabetic records, they cannot fake the glycosylated hemoglobin (Hb_{A1C}) level, which is a measure of long-term glucose control. This is produced by the attachment of glucose to Hb. The measure of the glycosylated fraction gives the average glucose concentration over the lifetime of the Hb molecule (120 days, normally 4–6.5%).

In type 1 diabetes, patient education and motivation are crucial to the long-term prognosis. Good long-term control is pivotal for reducing the long-term complications of diabetes mellitus. Focus on risk factors for ischemic heart disease and always ask specifically about visual problems and foot care.

Complications of diabetes

Review the frequency of acute complications of therapy or hyperglycemia. For example:
- Hypoglycemic attacks.
- Diabetic ketoacidosis (DKA).
- Hyperosmolar nonketotic coma.

Have they required hospital admissions for any of these?

Ask specifically about symptoms suggestive of poor control. For example:
- Weight loss, malaise, fatigue.
- Polyuria, polydipsia (due to osmotic diuresis).
- Blurred vision (refractive changes in the eye).
- Balanitis, pruritus vulvae, thrush.

Macrovascular complications

Diabetes mellitus is strongly associated with macrovascular disease. It is imperative that any coincident risk factors such as hypertension and hyperlipidemia are identified and minimized. Check for symptoms related to the three main forms of macrovascular disease:

- Ischemic heart disease (ask specifically about chest pains, myocardial infarction).
- Peripheral vascular disease (e.g., claudication).
- Cerebrovascular disease.

Microvascular complications

Long-term disease is associated with relentless progression of microvascular disease. Good control is clearly associated with a decreased likelihood of microvascular complications. Early recognition may allow specific therapy to be instituted. Ask about the three main forms of microvascular disease:

- Retinopathy: ask about visual symptoms, laser therapy. Have they had a dilated eye exam?
- Neuropathy: paresthesias.
- Nephropathy: proteinuria and hypertension.

Other complications

Diabetes mellitus is associated with other complications, which may be multifactorial. Specific inquiry should be made about:

- Impotence: rarely spontaneously volunteered by the patient, but common. Always ask.
- Staphylococcal skin infections (e.g., boils, carbuncles).
- Gastroparesis (nausea, vomiting, early satiety).
- Foot ulcers: neuropathy and vasculopathy. Common manifestations include numbness, pain, and paresthesias. Ask "Do you feel like you're walking on cotton wool?" and "Do you know where you're putting your feet?"

Past medical history

Review the other risk factors for ischemic heart and cerebrovascular disease. Consider other possible autoimmune diseases (especially thyroiditis, pernicious anaemia, vitiligo, Addison's disease), renal failure, and systemic infections.

Drug history

Review the agents used to control the diabetes and drugs that may be related to complications (e.g., antihypertensives, angiotensin-converting enzyme inhibitors, statins).

Oral hypoglycemic agents

Consider whether it is appropriate for the patient to be on an oral hypoglycemic agent. Beware of metformin in the presence of renal dysfunction (metformin is contraindicated as it may cause lactic acidosis). Consider whether it is more appropriate to use agents that are hepatically metabolized or renally excreted.

Insulin

Review the form of insulin used (e.g., long- or short-acting). Assess whether the dose needs to be modified. Ask about problems at injection sites (e.g., lipohypertrophy, scarring).

Review the use of other medications that may aggravate diabetic control (e.g., glucocorticosteroids, thiazide diuretics). It may be possible to improve diabetic control by appropriate adjustment of another medication.

Family history

This is usually positive for patients with type 2 diabetes mellitus.

Social history

Review home circumstances. For example:

- Is the patient's eyesight good enough to see the insulin syringe?
- Does the patient have sufficient manual dexterity (especially if he or she has neuropathy) to monitor his or her own therapy?

Education and motivation are central to the long-term outlook for the diabetic patient. An appropriate diet is essential for improving the control of all diabetic patients, especially those who are obese. Help from a dietician may be indicated. It is particularly important that the patient understands the unacceptable risks of smoking.

Diabetes is a condition in which a "patient-centered" approach has been shown to positively influence outcome. In diabetes mellitus, patient education and motivation are crucial to the long-term prognosis. Good long-term control is pivotal for reducing the long-term complications of diabetes mellitus. Focus on risk factors for ischemic heart disease, and always ask specifically about visual problems and foot care.

Presenting features of thyroid disease	
Hypothyroidism	Hyperthyroidism
weight gain*	weight loss despite good appetite*
general slowness	
mental slowing, poor memory	poor concentration
anorexia	
cold intolerance*	heat intolerance*, excessive sweating
depression	agitation*, restlessness*
coma	
constipation	diarrhea
altered appearance	eye changes
	palpitations

Fig. 11.1 Presenting features of thyroid disease. Asterisks indicate the more common or discriminatory features.

Thyroid disease

Presenting complaint

Hypothyroidism and hyperthyroidism may present in many ways, and form part of the differential diagnosis of a variety of disorders. Some of the more common presentations are shown in Fig. 11.1. A high index of suspicion may be needed to diagnose these conditions because presentation is often nonspecific.

Detailed history
Hyperthyroidism

Ask about symptoms of hyperthyroidism. Inquire specifically about palpitations (see Fig 11.1).

The common causes of atrial fibrillation are ischemic heart disease, hyperthyroidism, and mitral valve disease.

The following specific features may suggest underlying Graves' disease:
- Eye disease (diplopia, proptosis).
- Goiter (ask about difficulty swallowing or breathing).
- Pretibial myxedema.

Hypothyroidism

Ask about symptoms of hypothyroidism (see Fig. 11.1), such as tiredness, general slowing down, and deepening of the voice. In particular, inquire about weight gain, fertility problems, menstrual difficulties, and cold intolerance. The symptoms are often insidious and not noticed by patients or their immediate family, but they may be observed by occasional visitors or primary care physicians.

Past medical history

Ask about:
- Other autoimmune disorders (e.g., diabetes mellitus, Addison's disease, vitiligo, myasthenia gravis).
- Previous partial thyroidectomy or treatment with radio-iodine if hypothyroidism is suspected.

Hypothyroidism and hyperthyroidism can produce a multitude of symptoms. A high index of suspicion is needed, particularly in the context of mental changes, palpitations, changes in weight, altered conscious level, or cardiac disease. The most discriminatory features from the history are cold and heat intolerance and weight changes despite contradictory dietary history. A relative may provide invaluable clues as the patient may not spontaneously report symptoms.

Also consider treatable causes of thyroid disease (Fig. 11.2) and the presence of ischemic heart disease in hypothyroid patients as thyroxine therapy will then need to be more cautious.

Drug history

Review the use and dose of antithyroid medication and thyroxine. Consider drugs that may aggravate symptoms (e.g., beta-blockers causing bradycardia in hypothyroidism). In addition, consider drugs that may interfere with interpretation of thyroid function tests (e.g., estrogens increase thyroid-binding globulin concentration). Thyroid-stimulating hormone (TSH) levels are usually needed.

Secondary causes of thyroid disease	
Hypothyroidism	**Hyperthyroidism**
dietary iodine deficiency	
antithyroid drugs used at inappropriate dose or on resolution of hyperthyroid state	over-dosage with thyroxine
post-thyroid surgery	
radio-iodine therapy	thyroid carcinoma (rare)
tumor infiltration (rare)	TSH-secreting tumors (rare)
hypopituitarism	acute thyroiditis (e.g., infective, autoimmune)
post-subacute thyroiditis	

Fig. 11.2 Secondary causes of thyroid disease. TSH, thyroid-stimulating hormone.

Review of systems

A detailed screen of systemic symptoms is essential as many features are nonspecific. It is often fruitful to concentrate on psychological changes (e.g., symptoms of depression).

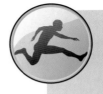

Try to assess thyroid status clinically in treated patients because biochemical tests lag behind therapeutic responses by several weeks.

PHYSICAL EXAMINATION

12. Introduction to Physical Examination

Overview

This section of the book is divided into the individual systems of the body. The first part of each chapter describes the routine examination of that system. The second part illustrates the process described above in practice by providing examples of pathologies or presentations related to the system. These examples are intended to provide a skeleton for the student's examination, illustrating the important features. It is important to get as much feedback as possible on your examination technique. Take every opportunity for someone more experienced to be present, watch what you are doing, and give you constructive feedback.

Setting

A good physical examination relies upon a cooperative patient and a well-lit room. It is important to engender an atmosphere of trust and professionalism during the history taking and to explain the steps of the examination appropriately and, if necessary, what information you hope to elicit from the process. This approach helps to avoid any misunderstanding and reassures the patient, taking away some of the mysticism that may surround the doctor–patient relationship.

Start each examination by washing your hands. It is important to be sensitive to the patient. It is always appropriate for a chaperone to be present; however, it may be inappropriate for the patient's partner to be in the room during the examination.

The patient must be appropriately positioned, comfortable, and in a well-lit, warm room. Insure that there is adequate privacy. Drape the patient appropriately. It is clearly unacceptable for a semiclad patient to be examined on a table without curtains if the door to the examination room is potentially going to be opened without warning or for the patient to be examined in a hospital room without curtains pulled round.

Examination routine

Although the examination is described as a separate process from the history, a good assessment should start as soon as the patient walks into the examination room (Fig. 12.1). There are countless other observations that can be made, and a rapid inspection of the patient will put the subsequently elicited history into context. For example, does the patient look ill or well? Have they apparently lost weight? Are there any obvious facial features, such as the staring eyes of thyrotoxicosis or yellow sclera of jaundice?

The examination, like the history, should be performed in a systematic manner, but again it is vital to be aware of the differential diagnosis as each sign is elicited. It is also important to think about what you expect to find from the history—it is easier to find something if you know what you are looking for. In many clinical examinations, including OSCEs, you may be asked to describe what you are doing and why, so it is a good idea to get into the habit. However, it is also necessary to keep an inquiring mind, as it is not difficult to convince yourself you have found the sign(s) that you expected, when in fact they are not actually present!

Once again the process is active. The examination routine usually follows a strict order. For most systems, the order of examination is as follows:
- Inspection.
- Palpation.
- Percussion.
- Auscultation.

Or in orthopedics:
- Look.
- Feel.
- Move.

The most important component of the examination is inspection.

Points to consider when the patient walks into the room
Does the patient look ill or in pain?
Is the patient cachectic or overweight?
What is the patient's ethnic cultural background?
Does the patient have a normal gait?
Is the patient short of breath on walking into the examination room?
Does the patient require help to get out of a chair?

Fig. 12.1 Points to consider when the patient walks into the room.

Examining a system

When examining any system, try to answer the following three questions.

What is the pathology?

This process requires interpretation of the physical signs so that a deviation from normality can be recognized and the individual signs integrated.

What is the etiology of the pathological process?

It is not enough to identify that a patient has a pleural effusion. An attempt should be made to find the underlying cause (e.g., lymphadenopathy and hepatomegaly suggesting malignancy, a third heart sound and elevated jugular venous pressure suggesting heart failure and fluid overload).

What are the severity and functional impact on the patient?

For example, severe aortic stenosis is an indication for valve replacement. This may be assessed clinically by measuring the pulse pressure and noting the presence of a slow-rising pulse.

Physical signs

Many physical signs are subtle, or simply represent a variation in the normal. It is essential that the doctor has an appreciation of the wide range of normality so that any signs can be placed into context. There are no shortcuts. To gain this ability requires practice.

13. Cardiovascular Examination

Examination routine

As with all examinations, the cardiovascular examination follows the format of inspection, palpation, percussion, and auscultation. Many cardiovascular pathologies produce multiple signs, which when integrated allow assessment of the severity and etiology of the lesion. It is particularly important to perform the examination in a systematic manner so that physical signs can be put into context with each other.

Patient exposure and position

Insure adequate lighting. The patient should be comfortable, seated at 45° to the horizontal, and stripped to the waist. Female patients should remove their bra. (It is difficult auscultating through clothing!) Provide a drape because the patient may wish to remain covered until examination of the precordium.

General inspection

In all systems, the specific examination should be preceded by an inspection of the patient. Vital clues are often found.

It is essential to know in advance what you are looking for, or it will not be found! Prepare a mental checklist. The whole process need take only a few seconds.

General features

Note any obvious features on general observation, including:
- Age, sex, general health.
- Body habitus (obese or cachectic).
- Breathlessness (observe the effort required to climb onto the exam table).

- Position in bed (is the patient comfortable, or does he/she seem to need to sit up or forward?).

Listen for any clicks of prosthetic heart valves. Inspection can then be performed from the head downward.

Eyes

A brief inspection will reveal abnormalities such as arcus senilis (significant in young adults, suggesting hypercholesterolemia) or xanthelasma (suggestive of hyperlipidemia). The patient may be obviously jaundiced.

Face

Look for evidence of cyanosis, particularly around the lips or under the tongue, or plethora (e.g., due to superior vena cava obstruction, polycythemia). The patient may have a typical facies for a pathological process, for example, malar flush (mitral stenosis).

Always inspect the mouth (dental hygiene in infective endocarditis).

Neck

Note any visible pulsations.

Precordium

Observe the shape of the chest for:
- Any obvious deformity (e.g., pectus excavatum in Marfan's syndrome).
- Visible collateral veins (e.g., in superior vena cava obstruction).
- Visible apex beat (e.g., left ventricular hypertrophy).
- Presence of any scars (Fig. 13.1).

Also look in the brachial and femoral regions for scars from cardiac catheterization.

Ankles

Briefly look for swelling suggestive of peripheral edema. This can be confirmed by later examination.

Adequate inspection is neglected at your peril! If it is omitted, simple diagnoses can be easily overlooked. It also helps to anticipate subsequently elicited physical signs and to put them in perspective.

Specific examination
Specific examination can now be performed.

Hands
Careful examination of the hands often reveals clues of underlying cardiovascular disease. Feel the temperature, and look for peripheral cyanosis. Note the shape of the hands (e.g., arachnodactyly in Marfan's syndrome).

Clubbing
The cardinal feature of clubbing is loss of angle of the nailfold. Other features include increased convex curvature in both a longitudinal and transverse plane, increased fluctuation of the nailbed, and swelling of the terminal phalanx (Fig. 13.2). Remember to look at both hands. Clubbing can rarely be detected in the toes. Hold the nail up to the plane of your eyes to facilitate detection. Although a nonspecific sign, its presence should alert the physician to underlying disease (Fig. 13.3).

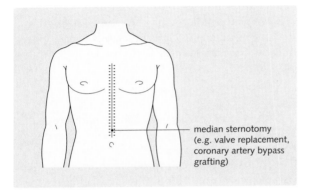

Fig. 13.1 Position of scars related to cardiovascular pathology on the precordium.

median sternotomy (e.g. valve replacement, coronary artery bypass grafting)

New-onset clubbing is highly significant. If it is detected, ask the patient whether he or she has noticed any recent change in the shape of the nails.

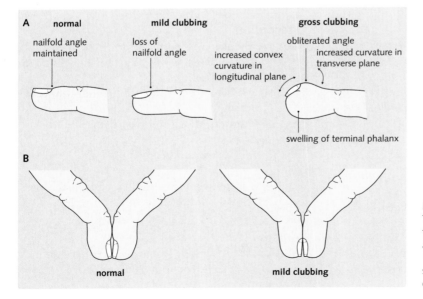

Fig. 13.2 (A) Features of clubbing. The cardinal sign is loss of angle of the nailfold. (B) If the patient is asked to place his index fingers "back to back," the diamond-shaped gap normally present is obliterated in early clubbing.

Splinter hemorrhages

These linear red or black streaks under the finger or toenails (Fig. 13.4) are a feature of a vasculitic process, but the most common cause is mild trauma, and a small number (e.g., about five) is normal.

Nailfold infarcts

Nailfold infarcts (Fig. 13.4) are also a feature of vasculitis, but more specific than splinter hemorrhages. They are often associated with other features of infective endocarditis (see Infective endocarditis).

Causes of clubbing	
System	**Disease associations**
cardiovascular	infective endocarditis* (late sign); congenital cyanotic heart disease; atrial myxoma (very rare)
respiratory	carcinoma of the bronchus*; fibrosing alveolitis*; chronic suppurative lung disease* (empyema, bronchiectasis, pulmonary abscess, cystic fibrosis)
abdominal	Crohn's disease (unusual); cirrhosis
familial	most common cause*

Fig. 13.3 Causes of clubbing. Asterisks indicate the more common causes.

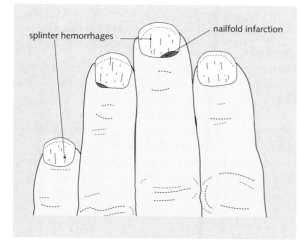

Fig. 13.4 Splinter hemorrhages and nailfold infarcts. If both lesions appear together, infective endocarditis or a vasculitic process is highly likely.

Capillary return

Apart from noting the temperature of the skin, peripheral perfusion may be assessed by capillary return. Light digital pressure to the end of the nail produces blanching. The speed of capillary return can be visualized. Poor peripheral perfusion can be easily detected. You should press on the nailbed for 5 seconds, and the return should take less than 2 seconds. Visible pulsation may be seen in aortic regurgitation.

Nicotine staining

Cigarette staining of the fingertips and nails may counter information given in the history.

Other signs of infective endocarditis

Look for other stigmata of infective endocarditis (rare). For example:
- Osler's nodes (tender nodules on the finger pulps).
- Janeway lesions (see Infective endocarditis).

Xanthomas

Lipid deposition may occur in tendons, skin, or soft tissues in some hyperlipidemic states. For example:
- Tendon xanthomas (especially of Achilles tendon, extensor tendons on hands): type II hyperlipidemia.
- Palmar xanthomas (skin creases of palms and soles): type III hyperlipidemia.

Arterial pulse

The arterial pulse may be palpated at various sites (Fig. 13.5). The pulse has various characteristics, which should be defined in each patient.

Presence and symmetry

Compare the radial pulsations synchronously (e.g., large vessel vasculitis, aortic dissection). Obstruction may delay the pulse. Check for radiofemoral delay, especially in hypertension (e.g., due to coarctation of the aorta). Assess the presence of each pulse, especially if there is embolism or peripheral artery disease.

Rate

Normal pulse rate is 60–100/min. Count for at least 15 seconds at the radial pulse. This may also provide an opportunity for additional visual inspection of the patient. The radial pulse rate may differ from the number of ventricular contractions per minute (e.g., apicoradial deficit in fast atrial fibrillation). Consider

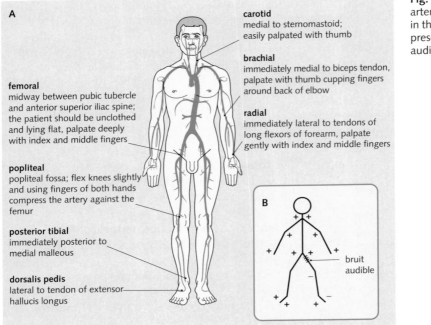

Fig. 13.5 (A) Location of the arterial pulses. (B) Typical notation in the hospital records (+, pulse present; −, pulse not palpable; bruit audible).

A

carotid
medial to sternomastoid; easily palpated with thumb

brachial
immediately medial to biceps tendon, palpate with thumb cupping fingers around back of elbow

radial
immediately lateral to tendons of long flexors of forearm, palpate gently with index and middle fingers

femoral
midway between pubic tubercle and anterior superior iliac spine; the patient should be unclothed and lying flat, palpate deeply with index and middle fingers

popliteal
popliteal fossa; flex knees slightly and using fingers of both hands compress the artery against the femur

posterior tibial
immediately posterior to medial malleous

dorsalis pedis
lateral to tendon of extensor hallucis longus

B

bruit audible

the rate within the clinical context (e.g., tachycardia in the presence of fever, hypovolemia; bradycardia in hypothermia, hypothyroidism).

Rhythm
The normal pulse rhythm is regular sinus rhythm. Any irregularity should be characterized and, if possible, confirmed by an electrocardiogram (ECG). Many arrhythmias are characteristic (Fig. 13.6). You should state whether the pulse is regular or irregular. If it is irregular, is it regularly irregular or irregularly irregular?

Volume
Pulse volume reflects stroke volume. This is best assessed at the carotid or brachial pulse. There is a wide range of "normal." It is important to practice on as many different patients as possible so that you can recognize when abnormal signs are present.

Some of the abnormalities of pulse volume include:

• Pulsus paradoxus. This is detectable in cardiac tamponade or severe asthma. A detectable increase in pulse volume is observed during expiration. Pulsus paradoxus reflects an exaggeration of the normal physiological changes in intrathoracic pressure and the influence of the diaphragm and interventricular septal changes during the respiratory cycle.

• Pulsus alternans. This is a sign of severe left ventricular failure. Alternate pulses are felt as strong or weak due to the presence of bigeminy.

• Coarctation of the aorta. As well as radiofemoral delay (described above), the pulse volume of the femoral pulse is usually noticeably reduced.

Character
With increasing distance from the aorta, particularly in sclerotic vessels, the waveform becomes distorted (Fig. 13.7), so volume and character should be assessed using either the carotid or brachial pulses. A picture of the waveform often correlates with the severity of valvular disorders. This sign requires considerable practice to elicit, so that the range of normality can be appreciated, and abnormalities put into context. Try to become used to the pulse character of the common pathologies (Fig. 13.7).

Blood pressure
Measurement of blood pressure is straightforward, yet it is often performed inadequately, with obvious implications for patient management.

Fig. 13.6 Common arrhythmias. In each recording the upper trace is the ECG and the lower trace illustrates a bar corresponding to each palpable pulsation. It is often possible to elucidate the underlying rhythm disturbance.

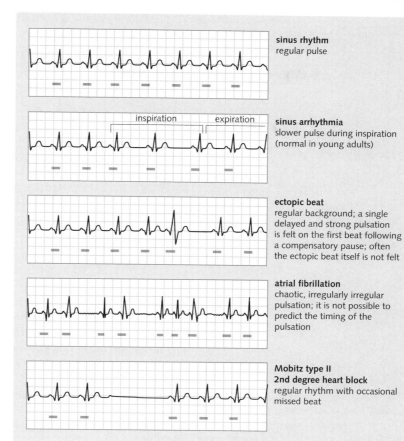

sinus rhythm
regular pulse

sinus arrhythmia
slower pulse during inspiration (normal in young adults)

ectopic beat
regular background; a single delayed and strong pulsation is felt on the first beat following a compensatory pause; often the ectopic beat itself is not felt

atrial fibrillation
chaotic, irregularly irregular pulsation; it is not possible to predict the timing of the pulsation

Mobitz type II 2nd degree heart block
regular rhythm with occasional missed beat

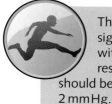

The blood pressure is a vital sign that should be elicited with great care and given the respect that it deserves! It should be measured to the nearest 2 mmHg.

As with other components of the cardiovascular examination, it is important to adopt a systematic approach:

- Allow the patient to relax. White coat hypertension is a real phenomenon.

- Make sure that the cuff is placed centrally over the brachial artery.
- Use a large cuff in obese subjects with an arm circumference over 30 cm—common cause of overestimating blood pressure.
- Deflate the cuff at a steady controlled rate—ideally no more than 2 mm per heartbeat.
- On deflating the cuff, note the point of the first audible sounds (Korotkov I), the point at which sounds become muffled (Korotkov IV), and the point of disappearance of sounds (Korotkov V, which is usually 5–10 mmHg lower than phase IV, but occasionally 0 mmHg). Most observers use phase V as a record of diastolic pressure because this produces less interobserver error.

Description	Waveform	Associations
normal		–
slow rising		aortic stenosis
collapsing (water hammer)		aortic regurgitation persistent ductus arteriosus

Fig. 13.7 Typical arterial waveforms palpated at the carotid pulse in different conditions. The waveform often provides important information about the severity of the underlying pathology.

Occasionally, additional blood pressure readings are indicated:

- Postural: for example, if the patient is on antihypertensive medication or has dizziness, or to assess hypovolemia.
- Comparison of right and left arms: for example, for aortic dissection, aortic coarctation.
- Repeated measurements: before diagnosing hypertension, always take readings on a variety of occasions.
- Comparison of the ankle/brachial ratio: for example, for aortic coarctation, peripheral vascular disease.

All these can be difficult to get as electronic measuring devices are taking over. You need to have a working knowledge of a manual sphygmomanometer and know where one can be found on the ward.

Neck
Arterial pulse
Follow the usual pattern of:

- Inspection: look at the pulsation (e.g., signs of collapsing pulse).
- Palpation: palpate the carotid artery specifically for volume and character.
- Auscultation: auscultate for the presence of a carotid bruit.

Venous pulse
Assessment of the jugular venous waveform is of fundamental importance to the cardiovascular examination (Fig. 13.8). There are no valves between the right atrium and internal jugular vein, which is readily distensible. Therefore, it can act as a manometer reflecting the filling pressure of the right heart. Examine the height of the wave. The jugular venous pressure (JVP) is measured as the vertical height of the column of blood in the internal jugular vein above the sternal angle (Fig. 13.9).

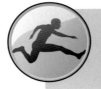

Assessment of the JVP should not be neglected. It is the most direct assessment of the filling pressure of the right heart.

Fig. 13.8 Characteristics of the jugular venous waveform and arterial pulse in the neck.

Characteristics of the jugular venous waveform and arterial pulse in the neck	
Jugular venous pulse	**Carotid pulse**
most prominent deflection is inward	most prominent deflection is outward
in sinus rhythm, two deflections for each beat	only one deflection for each beat
height of the wave changes with posture	height is independent of posture
temporary elevation of wave following pressure over the right costal margin (hepatojugular reflux)	constant
can usually be eliminated by light digital pressure over the clavicles	still present after light pressure
not palpable (in absence of tricuspid regurgitation)	palpable

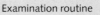

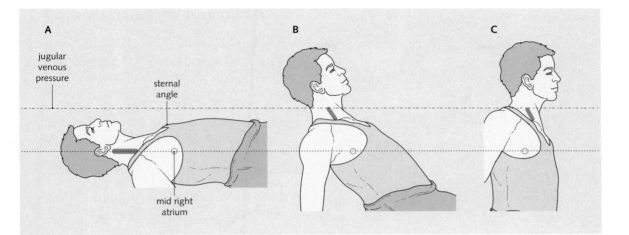

Fig. 13.9 The jugular venous pressure (JVP) is recorded as the vertical height of the visible waveform above the sternal angle. The pressure is fixed, but the anatomical position of the waveform varies according to posture. The jugular venous pressure is usually 2–5 cm.

The pulsation should be distinguished from arterial pulsation (Fig. 13.10). If it is not visible, the pressure may be:

- Too low (e.g., in hypovolemia). Lay the patient flat, test the hepatojugular reflux.
- Too high (e.g., in right ventricular infarction, volume overload). Sit the patient upright.

Note the character of the waveform. A basic appreciation of the normal jugular venous waveform is needed (Fig. 13.10). Assessment of the waveform requires considerable skill and experience. Unfortunately, there are no shortcuts. Assessment may give clues to pathologies such as tricuspid regurgitation (giant v waves), atrial fibrillation (no atrial systole, so only one component), or complete heart block (cannon waves).

Precordium

Although this is the meat of the cardiovascular examination, clues to underlying pathology should have been derived from the peripheral examination. Follow a strict examination routine. Remember that palpation should precede auscultation.

Apex beat

The apex beat is the most downward and outward position where the cardiac impulse is palpable. Define the following.

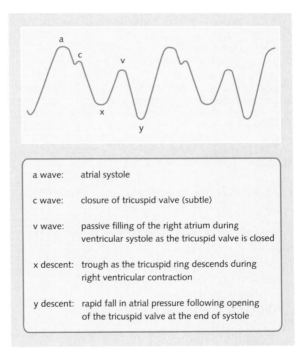

a wave:	atrial systole
c wave:	closure of tricuspid valve (subtle)
v wave:	passive filling of the right atrium during ventricular systole as the tricuspid valve is closed
x descent:	trough as the tricuspid ring descends during right ventricular contraction
y descent:	rapid fall in atrial pressure following opening of the tricuspid valve at the end of systole

Fig. 13.10 The components of the jugular venous waveform. In practice, the c wave is not usually visible. It is only by understanding the normal waveform that pathognomonic signs such as cannon waves and giant v waves can be recognized.

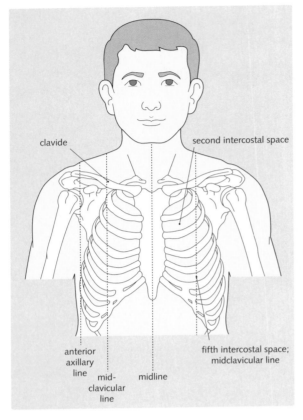

clavide

second intercostal space

anterior
axillary
line
    mid-
clavicular
   line

midline

fifth intercostal space;
midclavicular line

Fig. 13.11 Surface anatomy of the apex beat. It is defined in relation to the intercostal space and imaginary vertical lines related to the clavicle and axilla. The normal apex beat is within the 5th intercostal space in the midclavicular line.

Position The normal apex beat is within the 5th intercostal space in the midclavicular line (Fig. 13.11). A displaced apex beat usually implies volume overload of the left ventricle.

Character Check the character of the beat. For example:
- Forceful, "sustained," "heaving": left ventricular hypertrophy.
- Tapping: mitral stenosis.
- Thrusting: volume overload.

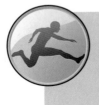

Be careful when describing the arterial pulse, apex beat, or heart murmurs, as certain terms often imply specific diagnoses.

Palpate the rest of the precordium

Note the presence of:
- Heaves—use either the palm or the medial aspect of the hand; right ventricular hypertrophy may cause a left parasternal lifting sensation.
- Thrills: palpable murmurs (especially in aortic stenosis) feel like a fly trapped in one's hands.
- Palpable heart sounds. For example, 1st heart sound in mitral stenosis felt as a "tap" at the apex.

Auscultation

Resist the temptation to auscultate until the rest of the examination routine is completed. It is much easier to auscultate when the sounds can be put into context with the rest of the examination.

An understanding of the cardiac cycle is essential when interpreting findings (Fig. 13.12). To begin with, time what you hear to the patient's pulse, as this helps in determining what you are listening to (Fig. 13.13). You will not pass or fail solely on what you hear. It is only part of the examination. Consider the most useful regions for auscultation (Fig. 13.14).

Listen in a systematic manner. In each region listen for:
- The first heart sound (immediately precedes systole).
- The second heart sound.
- Murmurs during systole.
- "The absence of silence," usually a murmur, during diastole.
- Any extra sounds (e.g., clicks, snaps).

If a murmur is heard, characterize its features as follows:
- Volume (Fig. 13.15).
- Onset: for example, presystolic, early systolic.
- Pattern: for example, crescendo–decrescendo pattern of aortic stenosis.
- Termination: compare the early systolic murmur of aortic stenosis and systolic murmur of mitral regurgitation.

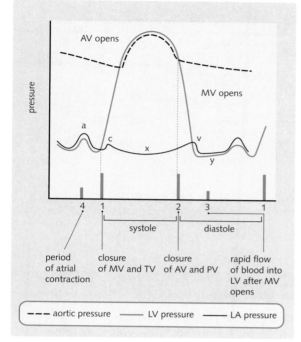

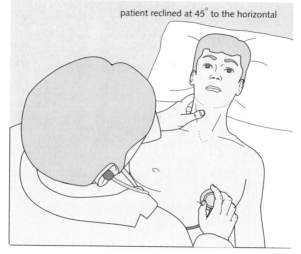

Fig. 13.13 It is essential to listen to the cardiac sounds while timing their point in the cardiac cycle by palpating the carotid pulse at the same time.

Fig. 13.12 The cardiac cycle. Systole starts at the point of closure of the mitral valve (MV)—first heart sound—when pressure in the left ventricle (LV) exceeds that of the left atrium (LA). There is a period of isovolumetric contraction before the pressure in the LV exceeds that in the aorta, at which point the aortic valve (AV) opens and blood starts to flow into the aorta. Following the onset of relaxation of the LV, the aortic pressure exceeds that in the LV and the aortic valve closes—second heart sound. The ventricle continues to relax until the pressure falls below that in the filled LA and the MV opens, allowing blood to flow rapidly into the LV. Atrial contraction precedes ventricular contraction, causing a presystolic accentuation of flow into the LV. (PV, pulmonary valve; TV, tricuspid valve.)

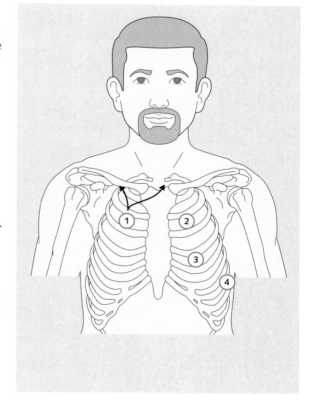

Fig. 13.14 Positions on the chest to auscultate for cardiac sounds. 1. 2nd right intercostal space (aortic area): mitral murmurs are very rarely audible here; if a murmur is audible, trace it toward the neck. 2. 2nd left intercostal space (pulmonary area): aortic regurgitation may be louder here. 3. 4th left intercostal space (tricuspid area): especially for tricuspid regurgitation, but mitral regurgitation and aortic stenosis are often also audible here; aortic regurgitation may be loudest here. 4. Apex (mitral area): listen specifically for mitral stenosis with the bell of the stethoscope; if a murmur is audible, trace it toward the axilla.

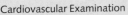

- Pitch: for example, low-pitched murmur of mitral stenosis.
- Location: where is it heard and where is it most audible.
- Radiation: for example, mitral regurgitation murmur radiating to the axilla.

Diastolic murmurs are often difficult to hear. Listen specifically for the "absence of silence" in diastole. Certain maneuvers (see below) need to be performed to augment the sounds.

To elicit aortic regurgitation, sit the patient forward and listen over the right 2nd intercostal space and left sternal border (LSB) in fixed expiration using the diaphragm of the stethoscope. To elicit mitral stenosis, roll the patient into a left lateral position and listen over the apex in fixed expiration using the bell of the stethoscope. Mild exertion may accentuate the murmur.

The different heart sounds are illustrated in Fig. 13.16.

Figure 13.17 is an illustration of a revision card detailing the order in which to conduct a complete CVS examination and what you are looking to find at each section.

Grading of the intensity of a cardiac murmur	
Grade	Intensity
I	just audible under optimal listening conditions
II	quiet
III	moderately loud
IV	loud and associated with a thrill
V	very loud
VI	audible without the aid of a stethoscope

Fig. 13.15 Grading of the intensity of a cardiac murmur. Don't ever be tempted to say a murmur is grade I or II. You aren't that good—yet!

Aortic stenosis

Diagnose the pathology

The features of aortic stenosis are illustrated in Fig. 13.18. The murmur needs to be distinguished from the ejection systolic murmurs associated with:

- Aortic sclerosis: this is common. The patient is usually elderly, and there are no hemodynamic effects.
- Bicuspid aortic valve: this is a common cause of an ejection systolic murmur in an asymptomatic young person.

Significance of different cardiac sounds		
Audible heart sounds	Timing	Cause
first heart sound	immediately presystolic	closure of mitral and tricuspid valves
second heart sound	end of systole	closure of aortic and pulmonary valves
third heart sound	early diastole	corresponds to period of rapid ventricular filling; normal in young fit people; associated with impaired LV function (especially raised end-diastolic pressure) (low-pitched, best heard at apex)
fourth heart sound	immediately presystolic	atrial systole; associated with noncompliant LV (e.g., hypertension); best heard with bell at apex
ejection click	early systole	opening of stenotic aortic valve
opening snap	early diastole	opening of abnormal tricuspid valve and especially mitral valve in mitral stenosis (well-defined short, high-pitched sound best heard with diaphragm at left sternal edge)
pericardial rub	systole and diastole	inflamed pericardium; coarse grating sound (like walking on fresh snow); accentuated by leaning patient forward; may be very localized

Fig. 13.16 Significance of different cardiac sounds (LV, left ventricle).

Cardiovascular examination	
General Inspection:	build, obvious pain/distress, features of Down's/Turner's/Marfan's
Hands:	anemia, cyanosis (poor peripheral perfusion), capillary refill, xanthomata – clubbing – loss of angle, 'boggy' nail, $\uparrow$longitudinal curvature, 'drumstick' – signs of endocarditis: splinter hemorrhage, Osler's nodes, Janeway lesions
Radial pulse:	rate (55-80 at rest), rhythm radioradial, radiofemoral delay (co-arc^n) – collapsing pulse (aortic regurg^n), bounding pulse ($\uparrow$HR, CO_2 retention, fever, LVF)
Brachial pulse:	character, volume – slow rising (aortic stenosis), collapsing/waterhammer (aortic regurgitation), – biphasic (aortic stenosis+regurgitation). Small vol (shock, $\uparrow$HR; mitral stenosis)
Eyes:	anemia, jaundice, arcus, xanthomata, conjunctival hemorrhage
Face:	central cyanosis ($\downarrow$SaO$_2$→blue mucous membranes) – malar flush (mitral stenosis)
Neck:	carotid pulse – separately – JVP – internal jugular vein – just medial to clavicular head of sternocleidomastoid • height of column above sternal angle. >4 cm if: RV failure, $\uparrow$vol, SVC obstruction a = atrial contraction, c = tricuspid value bulging into atrium, x = atrial relaxation, v = $\uparrow$pressure if atrial filling in ventricular systole, y = tricuspid opening in diastole. • waveform – double impulse No a wave in AF – cannon wave (giant a wave atrial contraction + closed tricuspid) – complete heart block, VT – systolic wave (c and v in ventricular systole) – tricuspid regurgitation
Pericardium	inspect chest deformity, scars, pacemakers, visible pulsations – palpate (i) apex-position (normal 5th ICS, midclavicular), character (tapping/thrusting), LV heave, thrill (MR) (ii) Ⓛ sternal border–parasternal heave (RVH), thrill of VSD (iii) aortic area–thrill of aortic stenosis, 2nd RICS (iv) trachea - mediastinal shift – auscultate–apex: heart sounds, added sounds, murmurs. Time a carotids – Ⓛ sternal border, aortic – pulmonary areas, Ⓛ axilla. Carotid bruits – Ⓛ lateral position – mitral stenosis (low pitched diastolic) – sitting forward, breath held in expiration – aortic regurgitation (Ⓛ lower sternal edge)
Lung bases:	pulmonary edema
Sacral edema:	ankle edema
Peripheral:	pulses, femoral bruits
Hepatomegaly, ascites	
BP	
Fundi	– silver wiring, a/v nipping, hard and soft exudates

Fig. 13.17 Card for cardiovascular examination.

- Subvalvular aortic stenosis: there is no ejection click.
- Pulmonary stenosis: this is rare. The murmur is loudest in the left 2nd intercostal space.
- Atrial septal defect: pulmonary flow murmur, fixed splitting of the second heart sound, and an associated tricuspid flow murmur.

Assess severity
Features suggestive of significant aortic stenosis include:
- Slow-rising pulse.
- Narrow pulse pressure.
- Displaced apex beat (suggestive of decompensation, unless there is associated aortic regurgitation).

Features of aortic stenosis	
timing of murmur	ejection systolic murmur
location	loudest over second right intercostal space, but often audible over the whole precordium
character	"harsh," often described as like a saw going through wood
radiation	radiates toward the neck
pulse	usually regular; may be slow-rising
blood pressure	reduced pulse pressure
apex beat	"heaving"
thrill	often present
other heart sounds	quiet aortic second heart sound; ejection click may be audible

Fig. 13.18 Features of aortic stenosis.

Consider etiology

The most common causes include:

- Degenerative disease (most common cause).
- Congenital anomaly.
- Rheumatic disease: now less common; look for associated valve pathology.

Aortic regurgitation

Diagnose the pathology

Aortic regurgitation is associated with a diastolic murmur, but there are other clues that indicate the presence of aortic regurgitation (Fig. 13.19).

The murmur of aortic regurgitation is often subtle. A specific attempt should always be made to listen for it. Sit the patient forward and listen with the diaphragm of the stethoscope in fixed expiration. Listen for the "absence of silence" in diastole.

Features on systemic examination include:

Features of aortic regurgitation	
timing of murmur	early diastolic
location	right or left intercostal space 2–4
character	usually quiet, "blowing," decrescendo

Fig. 13.19 Features of aortic regurgitation.

- Pulse: collapsing, high volume.
- Nails: visible capillary pulsation.
- Neck: head nods with each systole; vigorous arterial pulsation in neck.
- Blood pressure: wide pulse pressure.
- Apex: displaced (due to volume overload—bad sign), thrusting.
- Peripheral pulse: diastolic murmur over lightly compressed femoral artery.

Assess severity

Features suggestive of severe disease include evidence of cardiac dilatation and signs of left heart failure.

Consider etiology

Clues to the underlying pathology may be found as follows:

- Look at posture and arthropathy: ankylosing spondylitis.
- Look at eyes: Argyll–Robinson pupils associated with syphilitic aortitis.
- Look for high-arched palate, hypermobility, arachnodactyly: Marfan's syndrome.
- Check for other valve lesions: rheumatic fever, infective endocarditis.

Mitral stenosis

Diagnose the pathology

A particularly high index of suspicion should be raised in a patient with atrial fibrillation. Look for the classic mitral facies (cyanotic discoloration of the cheeks) and a tapping apex beat. The murmur is often very soft, and an attempt should always be made to specifically elicit it. Lean the patient on the left-hand side, and listen with the bell of the stethoscope in fixed expiration. It may be necessary to accentuate the murmur by exercise. The features of the murmur are illustrated in Fig. 13.20.

Assess severity

Look for features of left atrial overload and consequent left heart failure. For example:

- Cyanosis.
- Pulmonary edema.
- Hypotension (reduced cardiac output).

Look for features of right heart failure (raised JVP, peripheral edema, left parasternal heave due to right

Features of mitral stenosis	
timing of murmur	mid-diastolic (on opening of mitral valve); presystolic accentuation in the absence of atrial fibrillation (due to atrial contraction); if the mitral valve is mobile, the murmur is preceded by an "opening snap"
location	apex
character	"low-pitched rumbling"
other features	loud first heart sound; look for presence of mitral valvotomy scar

Fig. 13.20 Features of mitral stenosis.

ventricular hypertrophy). Atrial fibrillation occurs later in the natural history of the disease. The opening snap or onset of the murmur is closer to the second heart sound in severe disease as left atrial pressure is raised.

Consider etiology

Rheumatic heart disease is by far the most common cause.

Mitral regurgitation

Diagnose the pathology

Mitral regurgitation is commonly heard and produces a pansystolic murmur. It may be due to a number of different disease processes. Clues may be obtained before auscultation by the presence of atrial fibrillation (common, but less than mitral stenosis), a displaced thrusting apex beat, and occasionally a systolic thrill. Features of the murmur are illustrated in Fig. 13.21.

Features of mitral regurgitation	
timing of murmur	pansystolic (as systole starts from the closure of the mitral valve)
location	loudest at the apex; also often heard at the left sternal edge, but rarely in the aortic area
radiation	toward the axilla
loudness	usually easily audible

Fig. 13.21 Features of mitral regurgitation.

Assess severity

It is often difficult to assess the severity clinically, but a third heart sound and a mid-diastolic mitral flow murmur may be detected in severe disease. The severity is usually assessed by the symptoms and hemodynamic consequences.

Consider etiology

Mitral regurgitation may occur in any process that causes left ventricular dilatation and consequent stretching of the mitral valve annulus, as well as valvular pathology. The most common causes are:

- Ischemic heart disease: by far the most common cause.
- Rheumatic heart disease: relatively common in elderly patients, but now a rare disease; often associated with mitral stenosis.
- Infective endocarditis: look for peripheral stigmata.
- Papillary muscle rupture: especially after myocardial infarction.
- Mitral valve prolapse: common and due to ballooning of the posterior leaflet into the left atrium; it is associated with a midsystolic click and late systolic murmur.

Tricuspid regurgitation

Diagnose the pathology

Tricuspid regurgitation can often be recognized from the end of the bed by the observant examiner. It is usually due to primary left heart disease and secondary right ventricular pressure overload, so the signs may be due to a mixture of pathologies.

The jugular venous waveform shows characteristic giant v waves, and may cause oscillation of the ear lobes if the venous pressure is high enough. The patient often has signs of right heart failure with peripheral edema and occasionally ascites. If tricuspid regurgitation is suspected, the liver should be palpated for pulsatile hepatomegaly. In addition, the underlying cause should be sought.

The murmur resembles that of mitral regurgitation in many respects (Fig. 13.22).

Assess severity

Look for features of right-sided heart failure.

Features of tricuspid regurgitation	
timing of murmur	pansystolic
location	loudest at the lower left sternal edge
loudness	usually easily heard; may be accentuated by inspiration due to an increased venous return

Fig. 13.22 Features of tricuspid regurgitation.

Consider etiology

Tricuspid regurgitation usually results from right ventricular overload. The more common conditions predisposing to this are:

- Mitral valve disease.
- Cor pulmonale.
- Right ventricular myocardial infarction.

Primary tricuspid regurgitation may occur in:
- Rheumatic fever: rarely an isolated valve lesion.
- Infective endocarditis: especially in drug addicts (look for needle marks).
- Carcinoid syndrome: look for hepatomegaly, flushing, signs of pulmonary stenosis.

Infective endocarditis

Infective endocarditis may affect any of the heart valves. It often presents in a nonspecific manner and should be suspected in all patients with newly diagnosed valvular pathology or those with pre-existing valvular disease who develop pyrexia and malaise or a change in murmur.

Assess valvular pathology and severity

Define the valvular lesions and the hemodynamic consequences by a thorough cardiovascular examination.

Look for peripheral stigmata suggesting endocarditis

A complete systemic examination is essential as manifestations may arise from many systems. Features on systemic examination include the following.

Pyrexia

Fever is almost universal in infective endocarditis. However, it is often low-grade, and a single temperature reading may be normal. It is very important to follow the progression of fever through the course of the illness as a marker of successful therapy.

Nails (do not forget the toes!)

There are multiple stigmata of infective endocarditis in the hands. Many of these arise from an associated vasculitis. The following signs may be detected in the nails:

- Splinter hemorrhages. These are a nonspecific finding but common. They are suggestive of a vasculitic process. Although the presence is not specific for vasculitis, the occurrence of new splinter hemorrhages developing in the context of a new murmur and fever is highly suggestive.
- Nailfold infarcts. These are also suggestive of a vasculitic process. They are more specific but less common than splinter hemorrhages.
- Clubbing. A late sign and hopefully not present!

Hands

Vasculitic signs may also be detected in the hands:
- Osler's nodes. Do not forget the four Ps (painful, purple, papules on the pulps) of the fingers. They are rare, but enjoyed by examiners!
- Janeway lesions. These are rare transient macular patches on the palms.

Eyes

Fundoscopy is essential (especially in the exam setting). Look for Roth's spots, which are characteristic flame-shaped hemorrhages on the retina with white centers.

Splenomegaly

Splenomegaly is usually barely palpable if at all. There is little correlation with the duration or severity of the disease.

Hematuria

An immune complex nephritis is a common feature. Remember that urinalysis is part of the examination. Hematuria usually clears with successful antibiotic therapy. Occasionally confusion may arise as the long-term antibiotic therapy may precipitate interstitial nephritis (e.g., penicillins) or be nephrotoxic (e.g., gentamicin).

Fig. 13.23 Features of right and left heart failure.

Signs of right and left heart failure	
Right heart failure	**Left heart failure**
raised jugular venous pressure	third heart sound
peripheral edema	displaced apex beat (if volume overload)
ascites	pulmonary edema
hepatomegaly	tachycardia
left parasternal heave	cyanosis
cyanosis	cool, sweaty, pale skin (low output state)
tricuspid regurgitation	mitral regurgitation (due to volume overload of left ventricle)

Neurological signs

Endocarditis may present with neurological signs due to septic emboli in the brain. The elderly may present nonspecifically with confusion.

Consider etiology

Risk factors for infection may be elicited from the examination:

- Right-sided valve lesions, especially in intravenous drug abusers (*Staphylococcus aureus* and fungal disease more likely).
- Underlying valve lesion, usually present. *Viridans* streptococci are the most common agent; the most common predisposing valvular lesions are mitral and aortic valve disease, ventricular septal defect (VSD), patent ductus arteriosus (PDA), and coarctation of the aorta.
- Prosthetic valve.
- Dental hygiene: often the mouth is the primary portal of entry.

Heart failure

A simple diagnosis of "heart failure" is inadequate. An attempt must be made to assess its severity, functional impact, and etiology.

Establish the diagnosis and differentiate the features of right and left heart failure

Clues from the systemic examination are shown in Fig. 13.23. High output cardiac failure may also occur (Fig. 13.24). Not all of the features may be present; they depend upon the severity and underlying cause. Often the two conditions coexist.

Assessment of severity is usually dependent upon the history and the functional limitation imposed on the patient.

Consider etiology

The principal causes are:

- Impaired myocardial contractility.
- Arrhythmia.
- Volume overload.
- Pressure overload.
- Impaired filling.

Features of these conditions are illustrated in Fig. 13.24.

Myocardial infarction

Often there are no specific physical signs following a myocardial infarction (MI), but the physical examination can reveal complications and guide management, both in the acute setting and in the ensuing period.

Inspection

A quick visual inspection may reveal signs of pain or discomfort, necessitating better analgesic control. Assess peripheral perfusion; a cold, sweaty, cyanosed, pale patient suggests shock.

Features of different types of heart failure on systemic examination	
Cause of heart failure	**Features**
Impaired myocardial contractility ischemic heart disease	most common cause; may present as right, left, or biventricular failure; look for features to suggest other vascular disease (e.g., carotid bruits, signs of hypertension, etc.)
cardiomyopathy	look for systemic disease (e.g., amyloid, etc.)
myocarditis	look for signs of systemic infection; tachycardia is often a prominent feature; listen for associated pericardial rub
arrhythmia	common; often exacerbates underlying heart disease; may be able to detect arrhythmia from the pulse; aim to distinguish a primary arrhythmia from one consequent to poor myocardial perfusion
volume overload aortic regurgitation mitral regurgitation tricuspid regurgitation	look for signs of an underlying valvular defect; for left-sided lesions, identify a displaced apex beat
pressure overload hypertension aortic stenosis pulmonary embolus	slow-rising pulse; narrow pulse pressure; sustained apex beat right-sided signs associated with hypotension
impaired ventricular filling mitral stenosis cardiac tamponade restrictive cardiomyopathy	right heart failure; pulsus paradoxus; note jugular waveform

Fig. 13.24 Features of different types of heart failure on systemic examination.

Look specifically for complications

Always check for the presence of complications such as left or right heart failure and the presence of arrhythmias.

Left heart failure

Look for features of left heart failure such as:

- Signs of poor peripheral perfusion (impaired cardiac output).
- Low-volume pulse.
- Inspiratory crepitations at the lung bases.
- Gallop rhythm with third heart sound.
- Dyspnea.

These signs may indicate that the patient will not tolerate beta-blockade or may benefit from diuretics and angiotensin-converting enzyme (ACE) inhibitors.

Right heart failure

It is very important to recognize the patient with a right ventricular infarction. A disproportionately raised JVP in association with very poor peripheral perfusion, hypotension, and ECG signs are characteristic. Fluid balance in these patients is critical and demands central monitoring to assess left atrial filling pressure.

In the presence of shock and signs of right heart failure, always consider the presence of a posterior infarct, which may be subtle on the ECG.

Arrhythmia

Check the pulse carefully. Usually there is a mild tachycardia. The presence of a bradycardia suggests an inferior wall MI. The pulse may give clues to an underlying rhythm disturbance. For example:

- Heart block, especially following anterior wall MI.
- Atrial fibrillation (common).
- Ventricular extrasystoles.

These should be confirmed as the patient will have continuous ECG recording.

Subsequent examination

Particular features to assess include:

- Pulse rate (beta-blocker, primary cardiac rhythm disturbance).
- Blood pressure (e.g., cardiogenic shock, primary hypertension, new therapy with beta-blocker or ACE inhibitor).
- Signs of heart failure.
- Murmurs, especially the murmur of mitral regurgitation due to papillary muscle rupture and the long systolic murmur of ventricular septal defect.
- Pericardial rub.
- Psychological rehabilitation: often, the greatest morbidity on discharge from hospital is psychological. This should be recognized by eliciting the patient's concerns and treated early by appropriate education and reassurance.
- Signs of deep vein thrombosis, especially if there has been prolonged bed rest.

Examination routine

Patient exposure and position

The patient should be exposed to the waist in a similar fashion to exposure for the cardiovascular examination and seated comfortably on an exam table, inclined at 45° to the horizontal in a well-lit room.

 Remember inspection, palpation, percussion, auscultation.

General inspection

This should be performed systematically. As with other systems, think about which features you are looking for from the history before inspection. It is convenient to look first at the patient generally, and then to inspect specific features from the head downward. This process need take only a few seconds.

General features

Note the following features:
- Age and sex of the patient.
- General health and body habitus.
- Comfort at rest. For example, how easily can the patient climb onto the examination table?
- Respiratory rate. It is imperative that you count the respiratory rate. Don't make it obvious that you are observing the patient's breathing as this may influence the rate, especially in anxious patients.
- General environment. For example, in a hospital look on the bedside cabinet for sputum containers, nebulizers, inhalers, peak flow charts.

Head

Look for evidence of:
- Plethora (e.g., due to secondary polycythemia due to chronic hypoxia).
- Cigarette staining of hair and smell of cigarettes.

Chest

Note the presence of:
- Scars (Fig. 14.1).
- Breathing pattern (e.g., shallow or pursed lip and use of accessory muscles—sternomastoid, intercostals, abdominal).
- Chest wall deformity (e.g., pectus excavatus).
- Asymmetry (e.g., due to previous tuberculosis causing upper lobe fibrosis; kyphoscoliosis causing constrictive problems).
- Obvious tracheal deviation.

Specific examination

A more detailed systematic examination can now begin.

Hands

In particular look for the presence of:
- Clubbing.
- Peripheral cyanosis. If present, check for central cyanosis.
- Tremor. To demonstrate, ask the patient to hold out both hands with the wrists cocked back and to close the eyes. Then look for a tremor. The tremor of carbon dioxide retention is classically flapping in nature. If patients can see their hands, they can more easily control any tremor.
- Cigarette staining of nails and fingers.
- Painful swelling of the wrists (and ankles) is suggestive of hypertrophic arthroplasty due to squamous cell cancer of the lung.

Blood pressure and arterial pulse

A quick assessment of the pulse rate and blood pressure is useful. A hyperdynamic circulation may occur in carbon dioxide retention.

Head

An assessment should include specific inspection of:
- Eyes: to reveal, for example, Horner's syndrome (due to carcinoma of bronchus), jaundice, conjunctival pallor.
- Mouth: for example, tongue and mucous membranes may be cyanosed.

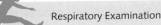

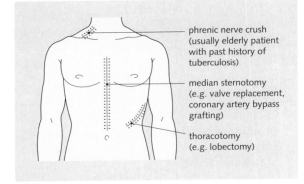

Fig. 14.1 Scars related to the respiratory system.

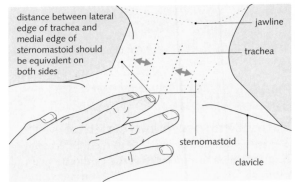

Fig. 14.2 Examination technique for assessing tracheal position. Place two fingers on either side of the trachea and judge the distance between the fingers and the sternocleidomastoid tendons.

Neck

Lymphadenopathy

Examine the cervical and supraclavicular lymph nodes. It may be easier to defer this part of the examination until the patient is sitting forward so that palpation can be performed from behind.

Tracheal position

Remember that this part of the examination is slightly uncomfortable (Fig. 14.2). The trachea may be shifted by pathology outside the chest (e.g., thyroid enlargement). Mediastinal position can also be assessed by determining the position of the apex beat.

> The tracheal position is often neglected by students, but this sign is of fundamental importance as it indicates the presence of a focal chest expanding (e.g., tension pneumothorax, massive pleural effusion) or constricting process (fibrosis, lung collapse).

Chest

Remember to examine the anterior, lateral, and posterior aspects of the chest. The routine for chest examination is straightforward, but the interpretation of signs requires experience as very often they reflect only a "qualitative" difference from the normal state. An appreciation of the range of normality demands practice! It is invaluable to have a more experienced observer who can provide constructive criticism of your approach and interpretation of signs with you while you are examining the patient.

Very few chest pathologies are manifest as a single abnormal sign. Rather, a constellation of signs needs to be interpreted in context and then integrated. The competent student will be constantly analysing the elicited signs and refining a differential diagnosis, anticipating how the next sign may modify the assessment. This highlights the importance of adopting an active approach to the examination.

It is a matter of preference whether the whole process is performed on the front of the chest and then the back, or whether each component of the examination is completed for the whole chest in turn, but the former approach is more comfortable for the patient and is preferred.

Inspection

If tracheal shift is noted, look more closely for asymmetry, especially scalloping below the clavicles suggestive of loss of volume of the upper lobe.

Palpation

There are three main components to this section:
- Assessment of mediastinal position.
- Assessment of chest expansion.
- Tactile vocal fremitus (TVF). (Vocal resonance is also discussed in this section for ease of explanation.)

Assessment of mediastinal position If the trachea is deviated, the position of the lower mediastinum can be assessed by determining the position of the apex beat.

Chest expansion Assess the degree and symmetry of chest expansion. Expansion should be assessed in the infraclavicular, costal margin, and lower rib region posteriorly. Place both hands around the lateral chest wall and approximate the thumbs in the midline but not resting on the posterior chest. Ask the patient to take a deep breath, and observe the displacement of the thumbs from the midline.

In practice, it is easier to detect decreased or absent tactile vocal fremitus and increased vocal resonance from the normal state. Hence, the two signs complement each other.

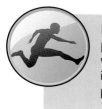

If there is unilateral chest pathology, the side of the chest with reduced expansion always indicates the side of the pathology.

Tactile vocal fremitus Place the medial aspect of the hand on the chest wall and ask the patient to make a resonant sound (e.g., say "ninety-nine"). The sound waves are transmitted as low-frequency vibrations, which are palpable. Different regions of the chest should be examined systematically, in particular comparing symmetry of the two sides. Make an attempt to define abnormalities in the upper, middle, and lower lobes. This requires an awareness of the surface markings of these lobes.

Vocal resonance This is included because it is complementary to TVF. Place the stethoscope on the chest wall and ask the patient to whisper "one, two, three." The distinct sounds are not normally heard, but a resonant sound as the sound waves are altered by transmission through the airways and chest wall. Once again, different regions should be examined systematically, comparing symmetry. Increased vocal resonance is termed "whispering pectoriloquy."

The degree of TVF or vocal resonance is dependent upon the transmission of sound waves to the chest wall from the large bronchi. It is therefore dependent upon the volume of sound generated and the conductivity of the lungs, which is dependent upon how close the stethoscope is to a large bronchus. It is:

- Increased in consolidation or lung collapse with a patent airway.
- Decreased in pleural effusion, pneumothorax, or collapse with an obstructed bronchus.

Percussion

Percussion is performed by placing the middle or index finger of one hand on the chest wall and hyperexpanding the proximal and distal interphalangeal joints so that the middle phalanx is closely opposed to the chest wall, and tapping it with the opposite index finger. This action should come from the wrist rather than being a hammering action; it should be just heavy enough to detect resonance. The percussing finger should be rapidly withdrawn after striking. Resonance is felt, just as much as it is heard. Percussion should be performed systematically as for TVF. Findings may include:

- Hyperresonance of the percussion note. This is often difficult to elicit but is present if there is more air in the chest cavity (e.g., pneumothorax, emphysema).
- A dull percussion note. This occurs if the lung tissue is replaced by solid material (e.g., consolidation) or if solid material is present between the chest wall and the lung (e.g., pleural effusion, pleural thickening). The note is said to be stony dull.

Auscultation

Breath sounds are produced by turbulent airflow and transmitted through the airways, lung parenchyma, pleurae, and chest wall. Changes in any of these structures can alter the sounds heard.

Auscultation is usually performed with the bell of the stethoscope as the patient breathes fairly deeply. Once again, it is important to compare findings on the two sides.

The aim of auscultation is to define:
- The quality of the breath sounds (Fig. 14.3).
- The presence of added sounds. As with cardiac murmurs, characterize the quality, volume, and timing.
- Vocal resonance (see above).

Description of quality of breath sounds		
Breath sounds	**Features**	**Examples**
vesicular breathing	progressively louder during inspiration, merging into expiratory phase with rapid fading in intensity	normal pattern
bronchial breathing	laryngeal sounds transmitted efficiently to chest wall if lung substance becomes uniform and more solid—blowing quality; pause between inspiratory and expiratory phases; expiratory phase as long as inspiratory phase	consolidation; collapse with patent bronchus; fibrosis
diminished volume	impaired conduction due to increased pleural/chest wall thickness or increased air acting as poor conductor	pleural effusion; pleural thickening; obesity; emphysema; pneumothorax

Fig. 14.3 Description of the quality of breath sounds.

Added sounds should be characterized systematically. Note the presence of the following.

Crackles (crepitations) These may be caused by secretions in the larger airways (e.g., in bronchitis, pneumonia, bronchiectasis). They are usually present throughout inspiration and may clear on coughing. Alternatively, reopening of occluded small airways during the later part of inspiration occurs in parenchymal disease (e.g., fibrosis, interstitial edema), where they tend to have a finer quality. Coughing will then have no effect.

Wheezes (rhonchi) These have a musical quality and usually result from narrowing of the bronchi due to edema, spasm, tumor, or secretions. They occur in:

- Asthma: polyphonic, mainly expiratory, diffuse.
- Bronchitis: may clear on coughing, may have an inspiratory component.
- Fixed obstruction: monophonic (e.g., due to bronchial carcinoma).

Pleural rub This sound is due to friction between the visceral and parietal pleurae in inflammatory conditions (pleurisy). It is often described as the sound of walking on crisp, newly fallen snow.

Other tests

Patients may have their own peak flow meter with them, or one may be available. Ask them to perform this test; watch and assess their technique. Ask the patient what the peak flow is normally; compare this value with today's reading and then with the predicted peak flow. Spirometery is available in many wards and examination settings. Get the patient to do this as well. With both of these tests, always have the patient make three attempts so that the best can be recorded.

Summary

At the end of the respiratory examination, it is important to take time to reflect on your findings. Remember that few lung pathologies have a single pathognomonic feature and that abnormalities are often a matter of qualitative judgment of deviation from normality rather than the simple presence or absence of a sign. The key to a successful examination is to be attentive and open to differential diagnoses from the start, so that physical signs can be anticipated rather than taking you by surprise. Figure 14.4 shows a review card for the respiratory system.

Pleural effusion

Diagnose the pathology

The physical signs can be anticipated from a basic appreciation of the pathology (Fig. 14.5).

Assess severity

Analyse the significance of physical signs:
- How high up the chest can percussion be demonstrated to be dull?
- Define the level of decreased breath sounds and reduced TVF.

Respiratory system examination
Undress to waist, sit on edge of bed. Look around—O_2, nebulizer, sputum pot, inhalers, spacer, etc.

General appearance	cachexia, respiratory distress, cyanosis/pallor/plethoric, etc. Sputum, temperature chart
Hands	clubbing, peripheral cyanosis, nicotine stains, asterixis (CO_2 retention trap)
Pulse, RR	central cyanosis, pallor, nasal flaring, cervical lymphadenopathy, jugular veins
Face	
Inspection of chest	RR, pattern of breathing, chest wall deformities, scars, chest wall movements
Palpation of chest	position of trachea, cricosternal distance, supraclavicular in RV heave
Chest expansion	assess upper and lower chest movement
Vocal fremitus	palpate chest wall as patient repeats "99"
Percussion	compare both sides, including clavicles, supraclavicular, axillae hyperresonant/resonant or normal/dull/stony dull
Auscultation	breathe in and out through mouth. Intensity—nature (vesicular/bronchial), air entry —bronchial breath sounds—high-pitched blowing, pause between insp and exp, consolidation/collapse —wheeze (rhonchi)—high/low pitch, insp/exp, monophonic/polyphonic effect of coughing —crackles (crepitations)—loud coarse/fine and high-pitched. Early insp—diffuse airways destruction (e.g., COPD) Late insp—diffuse fibrosis, pulmonary edema, bronchiectasis, consolidation —pleural rub—friction between pleura →localized creating, e.g., pleurisy, pulmonary infarction, pneumonia —vocal resonance—auscultate as patient says "99." Assess volume and clarity, whispering pectoriloquy.

Relevant CVS examination e.g., heart sounds, JV hepatomegaly, ankle edema

	Chest movement	Mediastinum	Percussion	Breath sounds	Visual resonance	Added sounds
Consolidation	↓ affected side	—	Dull	Bronchial	↑	Fine crackles
Collapse	↓ affected side	shift → lesion	Dull	↓ Vesicular	↓	—
Localized fibrosis	↓ affected side	shift → lesion	Dull	Bronchial	↑	Coarse crackles
CFA	↓ both sides	—	Normal	Vesicular	↑	Fine crackles
Pleural effusion	↓ affected side	shift away	Stony dull	↓ Vesicular	↓	—
Pneumothorax	↓ affected side	shift away	Hyperresonant	↓ Vesicular	↓	—
Asthma	↓ both sides	—	Normal	Prolonged exp	Normal	Exp polyphonic wheeze
COPD	↓ both sides	—	Normal	Prolonged exp	Normal	Exp wheeze, crackles

Overinflation	high shoulders, ↑ ant-post. chest diameter, using accessory muscles of respiration, limited chest expansion
Diffuse airways obstruction	wheeze, muffed cough, overinflation, costal margin moves in on inspiration, prolonged, expiration, early insp crackles, ↑ forced expiration time

Fig. 14.4 Review card for respiratory examination.

- How short of breath is the patient? (This may be altered by coexisting pathology and speed of onset.)
- Is the trachea shifted away from the effusion?

Consider etiology

Look for clues in the systemic examination:

- Palpable supraclavicular and/or axillary lymphadenopathy: malignancy.
- Hepatomegaly: secondary malignancy.
- Peripheral edema: hypoalbuminemia, heart failure.
- Third heart sound: left heart failure.

Consider the more common causes of pleural effusion (Fig. 14.6).

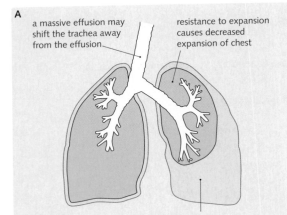

A

a massive effusion may shift the trachea away from the effusion

resistance to expansion causes decreased expansion of chest

fluid is not resonant (dull percussion note)

fluid surrounding the lung impairs transmission of soundwaves from the airways to the chest wall (causing ↓ TVF, vocal resonance and ↓↓ breath sounds)

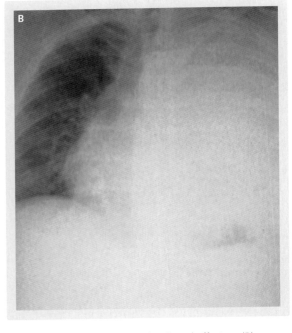

Fig. 14.5 (A) Physical signs of a pleural effusion. (B) Radiograph of a massive left pleural effusion. Note the tracheal deviation to the right. TVF, tactile vocal fremitus.

Pneumothorax

Diagnose the pathology

A small pneumothorax can be hard to identify, but index of suspicion should be high in tall, thin young adults with sudden-onset pleuritic chest pain and dyspnea. The basic clinical signs can be elucidated from basic principles (Fig. 14.7).

Assess severity

Most pneumothoraces do not cause hemodynamic compromise, but it is important to recognize a tension pneumothorax.

A tension pneumothorax is a medical emergency and should be identified and treated before requesting a radiograph. Treatment is immediate decompression with a 14-G needle placed in the second intercostal space in the midclavicular line.

Consider etiology

Most spontaneous pneumothoraces occur in previously fit young adults and are idiopathic. Look for underlying lung disease that may have precipitated the event. Consider the three major groups of precipitating pathologies, which are:

- Underlying medical disease (e.g., asthma or emphysema with bullae, carcinoma, tuberculosis).
- Iatrogenic (e.g., after central venous line insertion, especially subclavian line; intubated patient with positive pressure ventilation; after pleural aspiration or biopsy).
- Trauma (e.g., fractured ribs, surgical emphysema).

Lung collapse

Diagnose the pathology

Lung collapse may occur with a patent or occluded bronchus. The physical signs differ and may depend upon severity and underlying cause (Figs. 14.8 and 14.9).

Consider etiology

Consider the more common causes of collapse.

Extrinsic compression

The most common cause is lymph node compression due to tumor or tuberculosis.

Fig. 14.6 Common causes of a pleural effusion. The more common causes are marked with an asterisk.

Common causes of a pleural effusion	
Transudates	**Exudates**
fluid which has passed through a membrane	fluid containing proteins and white cells
left heart failure*	infection* (pneumonia, tuberculosis, empyema, etc.)
hypoalbuminuric states* (e.g., nephrotic syndrome, liver failure) fluid overload in renal failure	malignancy* (primary bronchial or metastatic) pulmonary infarction* subphrenic abscess
hypothyroidism Meigs's syndrome (right pleural effusion association with ovarian fibroma)	pancreatitis collagen vascular disease (e.g., rheumatoid arthritis) hemothorax

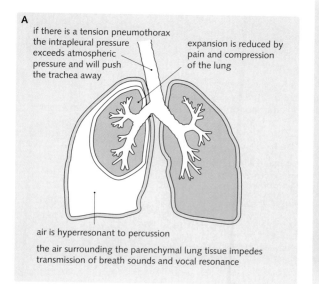

A
if there is a tension pneumothorax the intrapleural pressure exceeds atmospheric pressure and will push the trachea away

expansion is reduced by pain and compression of the lung

air is hyperresonant to percussion

the air surrounding the parenchymal lung tissue impedes transmission of breath sounds and vocal resonance

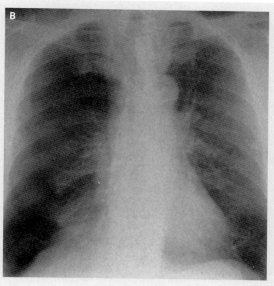

Fig. 14.7 (A) Physical signs of pneumothorax. (B) Radiograph of a right pneumothorax.

Intrinsic obstruction

Intraluminal obstruction may occlude the airway and cause distal collapse. The more common causes include:

- Tumors: look for clubbing.
- Retained secretions: postoperative, debilitated patients.
- Inhaled foreign body: usually apparent from history, especially right lower lobe—a medical emergency!
- Bronchial cast or plug: for example, due to aspergillosis, blood clot.

Consolidation

Diagnose the pathology

Consolidation implies replacement of air in the acini with fluid or solid material. The lung parenchyma is heavy and stiff but transmits sound waves to the chest wall more efficiently. In addition, the lower airways often collapse during expiration but may open explosively during inspiration when negative intrathoracic pressure is generated, producing crepitations (Fig. 14.10).

117

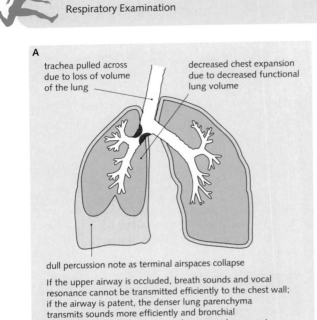

A
trachea pulled across due to loss of volume of the lung

decreased chest expansion due to decreased functional lung volume

dull percussion note as terminal airspaces collapse

If the upper airway is occluded, breath sounds and vocal resonance cannot be transmitted efficiently to the chest wall; if the airway is patent, the denser lung parenchyma transmits sounds more efficiently and bronchial breathing with whispering pectoriloquy may be present.

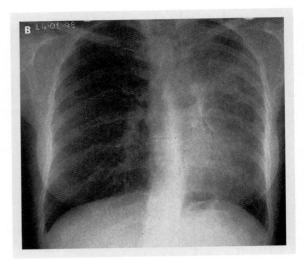

Fig. 14.8 (A) Radiographic features and physical signs of lung collapse with and without patent upper airways. (B) Radiograph of left upper lobe collapse: loss of lung volume is indicated by deviation of the trachea to the left, mediastinal shift to the left, and loss of volume of the left lung. In addition, note the classic veil-like opacification over the left lung.

Physical signs of lung collapse with and without patent upper airways		
Sign	**Patent upper airway**	**Obstructed bronchus**
expansion	always reduced on side of lesion	always reduced on side of lesion
trachea	deviated to side of collapse, especially upper lobe collapse	deviated to side of collapse, especially upper lobe collapse
percussion	dull	dull
TVF	usually normal or increased	decreased or absent
vocal resonance	whispering pectoriloquy	—
breath sounds	increased; bronchial breathing	absent or decreased

Fig. 14.9 Physical signs of lung collapse with and without patent upper airways. TVF, tactile vocal fremitus.

Consider etiology

The important causes of consolidation include:

- Pneumonia: most common cause, especially in classical lobar distribution.
- Pulmonary edema: may be cardiogenic or noncardiogenic.
- Pulmonary hemorrhage: for example, due to pulmonary vasculitis.
- Aspiration.
- Neoplasms: for example, alveolar cell carcinoma.

Look for systemic clues of the etiology:

- Fever, green sputum: pneumonia.
- Third heart sound, mitral murmurs, peripheral edema: cardiogenic.
- Nailfold infarcts, livedo reticularis, splinter hemorrhages: vasculitis.
- Clubbing: underlying primary bronchial carcinoma.

Differential diagnosis

Clinically, the main differential diagnosis is between pneumonia and pulmonary edema. This is usually apparent from the clinical setting.

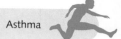

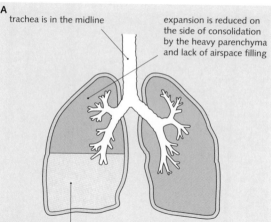

A

trachea is in the midline

expansion is reduced on the side of consolidation by the heavy parenchyma and lack of airspace filling

dull percussion note due to heavy parenchyma

the dense lung tissue transmits breath sounds and vocal resonance efficiently; crepitations are also present

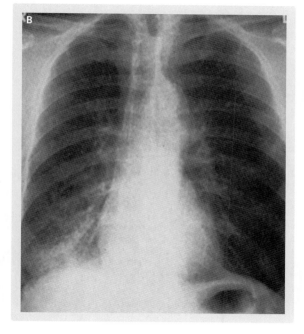

B

Fig. 14.10 (A) Physical signs of consolidation. (B) Radiograph of right lower lobe pneumonia.

It is more likely to be pneumonia if the consolidation is in a lobar distribution or unilateral (especially right-sided). In addition, a pleural effusion, raised jugular venous pressure, and peripheral edema are more common in pulmonary edema, but not diagnostic.

Lung fibrosis

Pulmonary fibrosis results in lungs that are rigid and resistant to expansion. The fibrotic disease often shrinks the lung, resulting in a constrictive process. The thicker parenchyma, however, transmit sound waves more efficiently to the chest wall. As with other parenchymal processes, the small airways may open explosively in inspiration, causing crepitations. The disease may be unilateral (e.g., tuberculosis) or bilateral (e.g., cryptogenic fibrosing alveolitis).

Diagnose the pathology

Distinguish between unilateral and bilateral disease. The tracheal position is most useful as often there is coexisting pathology (Fig. 14.11).

Consider etiology

The more common causes of pulmonary fibrosis are illustrated in Fig. 14.12.

Integrating physical signs to diagnose pathology

Figure 14.13 illustrates how the different physical signs elicited in the respiratory system can be integrated so that the basic underlying pathological cause can be identified. Remember that this is only part of the examination process. It is important to assess the severity of the pathology and its underlying cause so that specific therapy can be offered.

The importance of assessing expansion (to reveal the side of the pathology) and tracheal position (for expanding or constricting lesion) cannot be overemphasized.

Asthma

A diagnosis of asthma is usually apparent from the history. The aim of the examination is to assess severity, look for complications, and consider precipitating factors.

119

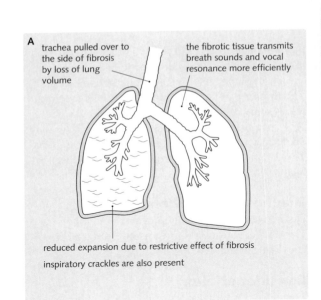

A
trachea pulled over to the side of fibrosis by loss of lung volume

the fibrotic tissue transmits breath sounds and vocal resonance more efficiently

reduced expansion due to restrictive effect of fibrosis

inspiratory crackles are also present

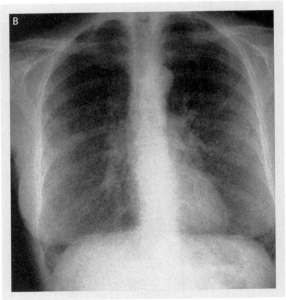

B

Fig. 14.11 (A) Physical signs of pulmonary fibrosis. (B) Radiograph of bilateral mid and lower zone pulmonary fibrosis.

Causes of pulmonary fibrosis	
Cause	Examples and signs
infection*	tuberculosis (typically upper lobe)
collagen disorder	rheumatoid lung (usually basal); scleroderma
extrinsic allergic alveolitis*	especially upper lobes
sarcoidosis*	look for erythema nodosum and other stigmata
radiation	look for radiation burns
drugs	busulphan, bleomycin, etc.
cryptogenic fibrosing alveolitis	rare; begins in lower lobes; look for clubbing
asbestosis	—
ankylosing spondylitis	upper lobes; rigid back; peripheral arthritis; aortic regurgitation, etc.

Fig. 14.12 Causes of pulmonary fibrosis. The more common causes are marked with an asterisk.

Assess severity

Severity is assessed by talking to the patient. If the patient cannot finish a sentence, he/she is having a severe attack and urgent help should be summoned. Use objective reproducible measures of severity and classify the attack as mild, moderate, or severe. Remember that not all of the features need to be present in a severe attack (Fig. 14.14). The essential parameters to assess are pulse rate, respiratory rate, peak flow rate, and (in hospitals) arterial blood gas estimate.

Other features of a serious or life-threatening attack include:

• Difficulty in speaking.
• Bradycardia or hypotension.
• Exhaustion.

Examination findings in the basic lung pathologies

Lung pathology	Tracheal position	Percussion note	TVF/vocal resonance	Volume of breath sounds	Added sounds
pneumothorax	normal (deviated away in tension pneumothorax)	hyperresonant (often subtle)	decreased (or absent)	decreased or absent	—
consolidation	normal	dull	increased	increased (bronchial breathing)	inspiratory crackles
fibrosis	pulled toward	slightly dull	increased	increased	inspiratory crackles
pleural effusion	normal (deviated away if massive)	stony dull	reduced or absent	decreased or absent	often crackles immediately above effusion
lobar collapse (patent airway)	pulled toward	dull	increased	increased (bronchial breathing)	—
lobar collapse (occluded bronchus)	pulled toward	dull	decreased	decreased	—

Fig. 14.13 Examination findings for the basic lung pathologies. Note that this refers to unilateral lesions. The expansion is always reduced on the side of the lung pathology. TVF, tactile vocal fremitus.

Assessment of severity of an acute asthma attack

Feature	Mild	Moderate	Severe
pulse rate (/min)	<100	100–110	>110
respiratory rate (/min)	<20	20–30	>30
peak flow rate	>75% predicted	50–75% predicted	<50% predicted
arterial blood gases	PaO_2 high/normal; $PaCO_2$ low	PaO_2 normal; $PaCO_2$ low or low normal (<38 mmHg)	$PaO_2 < 60$ mmHg $PaCO_2$ high normal or high (>38 mmHg)

Fig. 14.14 Assessment of severity of an acute asthma attack. In the hospital setting, arterial blood gases (ABG) form part of the routine assessment. Pulsus paradoxus, if easy to elicit, is useful, but often it is difficult—it is a waste of time making an inaccurate "best guess."

- Silent chest.
- Cyanosis.

Look for complications

Examine for the presence of a pneumothorax. This is the main reason for radiography in hospitalized patients.

Consider etiology

Look for signs of a chest infection, which is common. In older patients with new-onset asthma, look for nasal polyps, which are also associated with aspirin sensitivity. Also inspect for features of atopy, especially in younger patients (e.g., eczema, dry skin, thinning of lateral half of eyebrows from rubbing).

Asthma is potentially fatal. A rapid and objective assessment is essential.

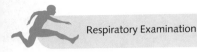

Lung cancer

Lung cancer is the most common fatal malignancy in men, and its incidence in women is on the increase. It can present in many ways and show many features on examination.

Inspection
Look for clues such as:
- Cachexia (common).
- Scar from lobectomy.
- Radiotherapy burn on chest wall.

Hands
There are often signs in the hands as follows:
- Clubbing: may predate clinical diagnosis.
- Clues to smoking history: nicotine staining on nails.
- Hypertrophic pulmonary osteoarthropathy (HPOA): pain and swelling of the wrists, especially with small cell carcinoma.

Face
Horner's syndrome (small pupil, partial ptosis, enophthalmos, anhidrosis) due to invasion of the sympathetic ganglion T1 by direct spread) may be a feature of upper lobe disease.

Neck
Palpate for a supraclavicular lymph node. Look for features of superior vena cava obstruction (swollen face and neck, plethora, dilated veins over trunk).

Chest
Look for features of:
- Pleural effusion (common).
- Loss of lung volume due to lobar or lung collapse.

Evidence of spread
Direct spread
Examine specifically for other features of direct spread:
- Pancoast's tumor—apical tumor invading the lower brachial plexus (especially C8, T1, T2) causing sensory loss, wasting, and weakness of the small muscles of the hand.
- Phrenic nerve: diaphragmatic palsy.
- Pericardium: effusion (look for features to suggest tamponade).

Metastatic spread
Examine for features of metastatic spread. For example:
- Hepatomegaly.
- Focal neurological signs due to cerebral metastases.
- Localized bony tenderness.

15. Abdominal Examination

Examination routine

A thorough abdominal examination is fundamental to both surgical and medical clerkship, but the emphasis clearly changes according to the presenting complaint.

Patient exposure and position

Insure good lighting. Patients should be undressed so that a view of the whole abdomen (from nipple to knees) can be obtained. Provide a drape for warmth and modesty. Lay the patient flat on the exam table with a single pillow behind the head (this may not always be possible—if, for example, the patient has orthopnea or musculoskeletal abnormalities), with arms by the side. If patients are unable to fully relax their abdomen, ask them to flex their hips to 45° and knees to 90° (Fig. 15.1).

The key is to have a relaxed patient. You will be able to elicit signs more easily if the patient is comfortable.

General inspection

Observe the general appearance of the patient. Time spent at this stage is invaluable. Take at least 10 seconds, making a mental checklist. For example:

- Is the patient comfortable or distressed at rest?
- Is there any obvious pain?
- Is there any cachexia, pallor, jaundice, abnormal skin pigmentation, distension, or other obvious signs?

A rapid but systematic survey of the patient should ensue.

Hands

Careful examination of the hands is fundamental to the abdominal examination and may yield vital clues of underlying abdominal disease.

If asked to examine the abdominal system, always start by looking at the hands.

Note the presence of:

- Metabolic flap (asterixis). This may indicate hepatic encephalopathy (or carbon dioxide retention and uremia).
- Signs of chronic liver disease. Inspect and palpate both hands for the presence of Dupuytren's contracture, palmar erythema, leuconychia (white nails), spider nevi, and clubbing.
- Anemia. If the patient is profoundly anemic, palmar skin creases may be pale. Koilonychia (spoon-shaped nails) suggests iron deficiency anemia.

Eyes

Inspect the sclerae for jaundice and the lower eyelid for anemia.

Jaundice is easily overlooked. It is harder to detect in artificial lighting.

Face

Note abnormal pigmentation around the lips or angular stomatitis, which occurs in many medical conditions, especially iron deficiency anemia, malabsorption, and oral infections.

Oral cavity

Inspect the oral cavity and tongue for:

- Ulceration (e.g., due to inflammatory bowel disease, chemotherapy).
- Inflammation.
- Oral candidiasis (e.g., due to antibiotic therapy, immunodeficiency, diabetes mellitus).

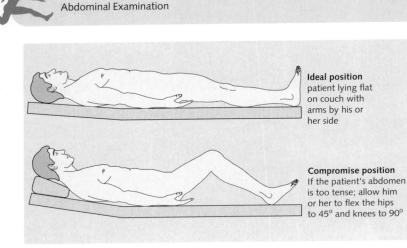

Fig. 15.1 Ideal position for examination of the abdomen.

Ideal position
patient lying flat on couch with arms by his or her side

Compromise position
If the patient's abdomen is too tense; allow him or her to flex the hips to 45° and knees to 90°

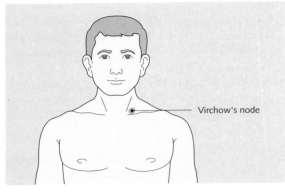

Fig. 15.2 Virchow's node is a palpable left supraclavicular lymph node. Troisier's sign refers to the presence of a palpable left supraclavicular node in association with gastric carcinoma. This node is easiest to palpate from behind.

- Halitosis (e.g., due to infection, poor hygiene, hepatic fetor, uremia, diabetes mellitus).
- Pigmentation (e.g., Addison's disease)

Chest wall

Note the presence of gynecomastia and spider nevi. The presence of more than five spider nevi is considered to be suggestive of liver disease. These characteristically blanche if the central arteriole is pressed.

Supraclavicular lymphadenopathy

Pay particular attention to the left side, and look for Virchow's node (Fig. 15.2). If present, is this Troisier's sign?

Exposure of the abdomen

Following general inspection, the abdomen should be exposed from the nipples to symphysis pubis.

Auscultation

Listen specifically for bowel sounds. The presence or absence of bowel sounds is important. Listen for 30 seconds before concluding that bowel sounds are absent. Much mythology has been generated about the quality of these sounds, but this should be interpreted with caution. Listen specifically for bruits over the aorta and renal arteries.

Inspection

Stand at the end of the bed and inspect the abdomen for:
- Symmetry (e.g., massive splenomegaly produces a bulge on the left side).
- Abnormal pulsation (e.g., due to abdominal aortic aneurysm).
- Shape (e.g., distension).

Remember the five Fs from Chapter 6.

Return to the right-hand side of the abdomen and actively inspect for the presence of:
- Scars (Fig. 15.3).
- Sinuses (e.g., due to retained suture material).
- Fistulas (e.g., due to Crohn's disease).
- Visible peristalsis (e.g., due to intestinal obstruction).
- Distended veins.
- Flank hemorrhages (e.g., due to pancreatitis).

Ask patients whether they are aware of any abnormal lumps or areas of tenderness. This may give a clue to the area of pathology. Ask patients to cough,

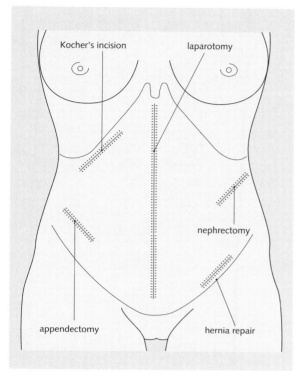

Fig. 15.3 Surgical scars on the abdominal wall.

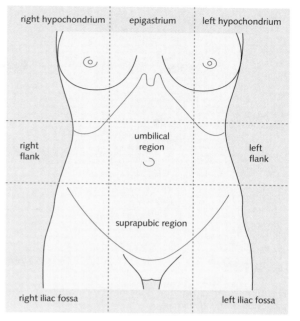

Fig. 15.4 The regions of the abdomen. It is helpful to be aware of these regions when palpating or presenting physical findings as this helps in the differential diagnosis.

observing pain (peritoneal irritation) and also the hernial orifices.

Palpation

Before palpating, ask the patient where the pain is. Warn the patient that you are going to lay your hand on the abdomen. Lay your hand on the point furthest from the pain and work toward it. The three stages to abdominal palpation are:

- Light palpation.
- Deep palpation.
- Specific palpation of the intra-abdominal organs.

Light palpation

Commence palpation at a site remote from the area of pain. All areas of the abdomen must be palpated systematically. Picture the abdomen in nine regions (Fig. 15.4). (Some people refer to abdominal quadrants as shown in Fig. 15.5.) This helps you to adopt a systematic approach to the examination and when presenting your findings.

Light palpation is performed to elicit any tenderness or guarding. Lay the hands and fingers flat

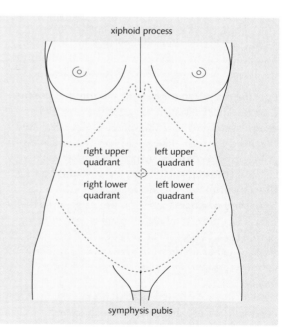

Fig. 15.5 The four quadrants of the abdomen.

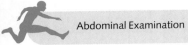

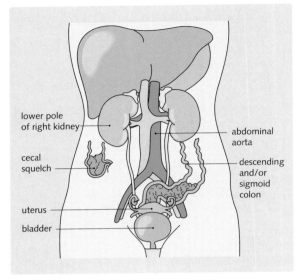

Fig. 15.6 Normal structures that may be palpable on deep palpation of the abdomen.

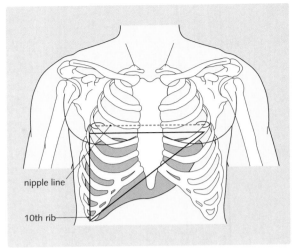

Fig. 15.7 Surface anatomy of the liver.

upon the abdomen and press very gently. It is essential to be as gentle as possible:

- To gain the patient's confidence.
- To prevent voluntary guarding (tensing of the abdominal wall musculature as light pressure is applied), which will mask pathological signs.

Deep palpation

Warn the patient that you will be pressing more firmly, and feel for any obvious masses (Fig. 15.6) or tenderness in the nine regions. If a mass is identified, determine its characteristics systematically.

Specific palpation of the intra-abdominal organs

Liver Always start in the right iliac fossa when examining the liver or the spleen as both expand toward this region. Place your hand flat with fingers pointing toward the patient's head (or alternatively to the left flank), and palpate deeply while asking the patient to breathe in and out deeply. Keep your hands still while the patient is breathing in as the liver edge moves downward on inspiration. If nothing is felt, repeat the process with the hand slightly higher up the abdomen, advancing a few centimeters at a time until the costal margin is reached.

The liver may be palpated in normal subjects, especially if they are thin or if there is chest hyperinflation (Fig. 15.7). If the liver edge is palpable, describe:

- The size of the liver (measure with percussion; in centimeters).
- Its contour (regular or irregular).
- Its texture (smooth, nodular).
- Any tenderness (see Hepatomegaly).

After this percuss outward to the superior and inferior borders of the liver.

Spleen The spleen is examined by a similar process as for the liver. Start in the right iliac fossa with fingers pointing toward the left costal margin and ask the patient to breathe in and out while advancing toward the left costal margin. If there is no obvious splenomegaly, ask the patient to roll onto the right side, place your left hand around the lower left costal margin, and lift forward as the patient inspires, while palpating with your right hand (Fig. 15.8).

A normal spleen is not palpable.

Kidneys The kidneys are examined bimanually by the technique of ballottement. The left kidney is felt by placing your left hand in the left flank below the 12th rib lateral to the erector spinae muscles and above the iliac crest with the right hand placed anteriorly just above the anterior superior iliac spine. During inspiration, the left hand is then lifted gently upward toward the right hand (Fig. 15.9).

The kidney may be palpable in thin normal individuals. The right kidney is examined with

126

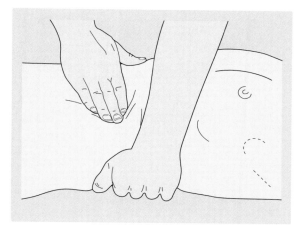

Fig. 15.8 Palpation of the spleen: initial examination. If the examination is difficult, the patient should be asked to roll onto the right side, push the spleen forward with your left hand and palpate with your right hand.

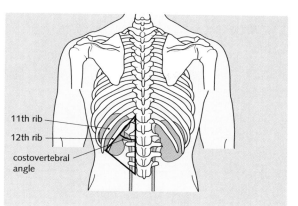

Fig. 15.10 Surface anatomy of the kidneys.

11th rib
12th rib
costovertebral angle

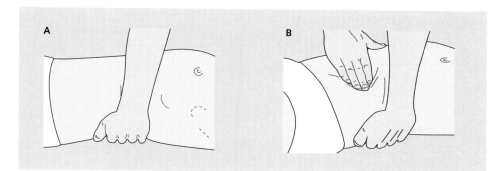

A   B

Fig. 15.9 Palpation of the kidneys.

the right hand posteriorly and the left hand anteriorly.

In normal individuals, the right kidney lies lower than the left (due to downward displacement by the liver) and is more likely to be palpable (Fig. 15.10).

Abdominal aorta   Palpate specifically for an abdominal aortic aneurysm (AAA). This is performed by placing the palmar surfaces of both hands laterally and with the fingertips positioned in the midline a few centimeters below the xiphoid process (Fig. 15.11).

- An AAA is both pulsatile and expansile (fingertips are pushed outward).
- A nonaneurysmal abdominal aorta is only pulsatile (fingertips pushed upward but not outward) (Fig. 15.12).

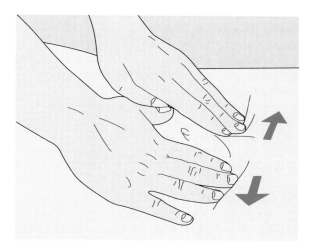

Fig. 15.11 Palpation for the abdominal aorta.

127

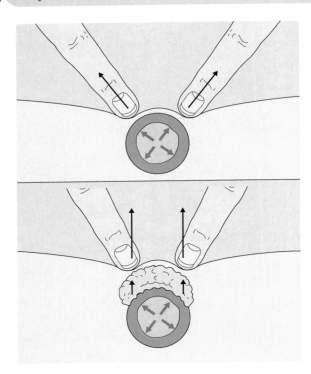

Fig. 15.12 Distinction between aortic pulsation and movement of an overlying structure. True pulsatility is indicated by outward displacement of the palpating hands.

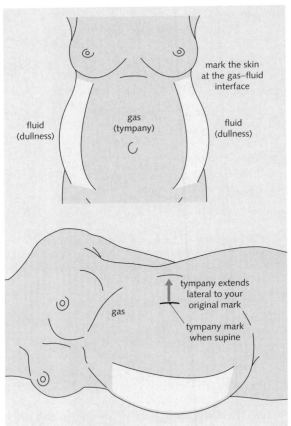

Fig. 15.13 Shifting dullness is a key sign of ascites.

Percussion

Percuss over the whole abdomen and particularly over masses. This is also a sensitive method for eliciting peritonitis. Specifically percuss for ascites by testing for shifting dullness. Percuss from the midline to the flank. If ascites is present, the initially resonant note will become dull. Note the point of transition on the skin, ask the patient to roll away from that side, wait a few seconds, and percuss over that area. If ascites is present, the initially dull note will become resonant (Figs. 15.13 and 15.14).

A complete abdominal examination includes assessment of:
- The hernial orifices. (See Chapter 17.)
- External genitalia. (See Chapter 17.)
- A rectal examination.

Rectal examination

The rectal examination is usually performed with the patient in the left lateral position, with both hips and knees fully flexed (Fig. 15.15). It is essential to explain the procedure to the patient and to be gentle!

It is usually possible to palpate lesions up to 6–8 cm from the anal verge. Before performing a digital examination:
- Inspect the anus, its margins, and surrounding skin.
- Look for skin tags, excoriation, prolapsed or thrombosed hemorrhoids, fistulas, fissures, abscesses, or ulceration due to an anal carcinoma.
- Ask the patient to bear down or strain. This may reveal the presence of a rectal prolapse or occasionally a polyp.

While performing a digital rectal examination, the sphincter tone should be assessed and any tenderness elicited.

Structures palpable during a normal digital rectal examination

Palpate anteriorly, laterally, and posteriorly. Note the following:

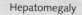

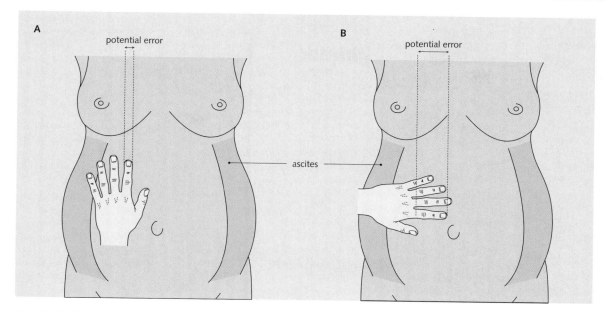

Fig. 15.14 Correct orientation of your hands is important when percussing the abdomen for the presence of ascites. (A) Correct positioning of the hand. (B) Incorrect positioning of the hand.

- Posteriorly: the tip of the coccyx and sacrum are palpable.
- Laterally: ischial spines and ischiorectal fossa.
- Anteriorly in males: prostate (smooth lateral lobes separated by the median sulcus). A prostatic carcinoma may be differentiated from benign prostatic hypertrophy by the loss of the median sulcus and possibly the presence of a palpable hard, craggy, irregular mass.
- Anteriorly in females: cervix through the vaginal wall and occasionally the body of the uterus.

The normal rectum may contain some feces. Always look at the glove after examination for blood or mucus. Melena stool has the appearance of sticky tar and an offensive characteristic smell. A rectal carcinoma may be palpable as a shelf-like lesion associated with blood on the glove.

Always wipe the patient after examination and offer further tissues.

Hepatomegaly

Identify the mass as the liver

The liver is palpable in the right upper quadrant. Hepatomegaly is not usually confused with other organomegaly, but the liver should be distinguished from an enlarged right kidney. The features of hepatomegaly include:

- Palpable below the right costal margin (in gross hepatomegaly, it may extend to the left costal margin).
- Downward movement on inspiration.
- Dullness to percussion.
- It is impossible to palpate above the upper margin of the liver.

Define the characteristics of the liver

It is often possible to palpate a liver edge 1–2 cm below the right costal margin. If the liver edge is palpable, it is important to confirm that there is true hepatomegaly rather than a low diaphragm (e.g., due to chronic obstructive airways disease).

The size of the liver may be confirmed by percussion in a sagittal plane recording the "height" of the liver. A normal liver is less than 15 cm. Record:

- Size of the liver. Once true hepatomegaly is confirmed, trace out the edge of the liver to define its margins. An enlarged right lobe (Riedel's lobe) is a normal finding. In the notes it is helpful to record accurately the size of the liver in the midclavicular line, midline, and, if appropriate, the left midclavicular line.
- Consistency of the liver (e.g., hard, firm).

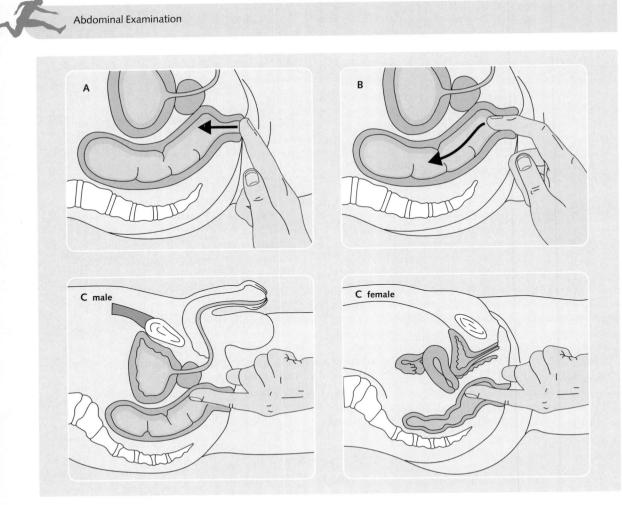

Fig. 15.15 The rectal examination. (A) Insert the tip of your index finger into the anal canal. (B) Follow the curve of the sacrum. (C) Sweep the finger around the pelvis, noting any irregularities, masses, or tenderness. Examine the glove on withdrawal of your finger.

- Definition of the liver edge (e.g., smooth, knobbly).
- Tenderness (e.g., engorged liver in right heart failure).
- Pulsatility (e.g., as in tricuspid stenosis).

Consider etiology

It is important to look for other features on systemic examination if hepatomegaly is found as they may give clues to the underlying pathology (Fig. 15.16). In particular look for:

- Signs of chronic liver disease (e.g., due to alcoholic cirrhosis).
- Splenomegaly (e.g., due to portal hypertension, lymphoma).

- Generalized lymphadenopathy (e.g., due to lymphoma, carcinoma).
- Jugular venous wave (e.g., due to right heart failure, tricuspid regurgitation).
- Features of underlying malignancy.

Assess severity

Look for features of hepatic decompensation. For example:

- Features of chronic liver disease (e.g., testicular atrophy, loss of axillary hair, gynecomastia, spider nevi, leuconychia). These features suggest that the underlying disease process is chronic.
- Signs of portal hypertension. Always specifically check for ascites and splenomegaly. Look for a

Causes of hepatomegaly	
Causes*	Features on examination
cirrhosis	features of chronic liver disease; features of portal hypertension; hard, irregular, knobbly liver common
alcoholic	common; look for evidence of alcoholic toxicity in other systems (e.g., neuropathy)
primary biliary	usually middle-aged female; pruritus common (look for excoriation); xanthelasma
hemochromatosis	skin pigmentation; gonadal atrophy; more common in men
α-1-antitrypsin deficiency	signs of chronic obstructive airways disease
secondary carcinoma*	hard, irregular, knobbly liver edge; systemic features of malignancy (e.g., cachexia, etc.); lymphadenopathy; signs of primary (e.g., palpable breast lump, etc.)
congestive cardiac failure*	raised jugular venous pressure; peripheral edema prominent; third heart sound; look for features of tricuspid regurgitation
infections (hepatitis A, B, C—rarely; glandular fever; cytomegalovirus; leptospirosis; hydatid; amebic)	features are usually apparent from the history, but look for generalized lymphadenopathy
lymphoproliferative disorder (lymphoma; leukemia; polycythemia)	splenomegaly; generalized lymphadenopathy; anemia or plethora; petechiae; etc.
miscellaneous amyloid polycystic fatty liver	splenomegaly; waxy skin; chronic disease; palpable kidneys; signs of uremia

Fig. 15.16 Causes of hepatomegaly. The most common causes are cirrhosis, secondary carcinoma, and congestive cardiac failure.

caput medusae (dilated collateral veins radiating from the umbilicus).
- Signs of hepatic encephalopathy. Check the patient's mental state (especially for level of consciousness and constructional apraxia; Fig. 15.17). Specifically check for a metabolic flap (asterixis).
- Jaundice.

Splenomegaly

Identify the mass as the spleen
A mass in the left upper quadrant is usually a spleen. It is not normal to be able to palpate the spleen. It must be enlarged 2- to 3-fold before it becomes palpable. It must be distinguished from the left kidney.

The characteristics of the spleen on physical examination include:
- Presence in the left upper quadrant.
- Upper edge not palpable.

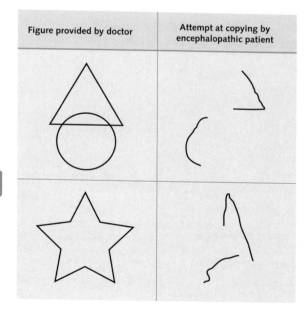

| Figure provided by doctor | Attempt at copying by encephalopathic patient |

Fig. 15.17 Hepatic encephalopathy is associated with constructional apraxia. Ask the patient to copy a simple figure such as a five-pointed star or simple overlapping geometric shapes.

131

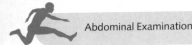

- Expansion toward the right lower quadrant.
- On inspiration, movement toward the right lower quadrant.
- A notch may be palpable.
- Dullness to percussion. The dullness extends above the costal margin.
- Not ballotable.

Assess spleen size

In a manner analogous to assessing the degree of hepatomegaly, it is important to measure the descent of the spleen from the left costal margin (Fig. 15.18).

Consider etiology

The more common causes of splenomegaly are illustrated in Fig. 15.19. In particular, note the presence of:

- Hepatomegaly: portal hypertension, lymphoproliferative disorder.
- Generalized lymphadenopathy: lymphoproliferative disorder.
- Size of spleen: massive splenomegaly is usually due to chronic malaria, myelofibrosis, or chronic myeloid leukemia (CML); a barely palpable spleen has a much wider differential diagnosis.

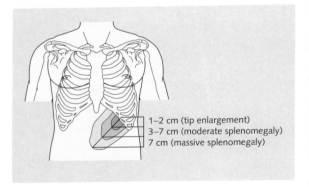

Fig. 15.18 Different degrees of splenomegaly.

1–2 cm (tip enlargement)
3–7 cm (moderate splenomegaly)
7 cm (massive splenomegaly)

Figure 15.20 is an outline of the approach to the abdominal examination.

Anemia

The causes of anemia are widespread. Remember the section in Chapter 6. The diagnosis is largely made from detailed laboratory testing and imaging investigations. However, it is essential that the investigation is focused, and this relies upon a systematic assessment during the history and examination.

Anemia is usually detected clinically if the hemoglobin concentration is less than 10 g/dL. The signs of anemia include:

- Conjunctival or mucosal pallor.
- Loss of color in the palmar skin creases.

The more common causes of anemia are:

- Iron deficiency anemia.
- Folate deficiency.
- Vitamin B_{12} deficiency.
- Hemolytic anemia.

However, these diagnoses are insufficient. An underlying cause still needs to be identified in order to provide suitable treatment and prognostic information.

Attempt to define the cause of anemia

A thorough systematic examination is essential. Clues may be found by considering the following.

General inspection

Inspect the face carefully. Look at the general health of the patient (e.g., cachexia suggests chronic disease), and note specifically any obvious disorders (e.g., rheumatoid arthritis). Some clues to iron deficiency and megaloblastic anemia are illustrated in Fig. 15.21.

Causes of splenomegaly		
Large (past umbilicus)	Moderate (to umbilicus)	Mild (just palpable)
Myelofibrosis	Chronic lymphatic leukemia	Portal hypertension
Chronic myeloid leukemia	Lymphoma	Lymphoma
Malaria	Portal hypertension	Rheumatoid arthritis (Felty's syndrome)
		Chronic lymphatic leukemia

Fig. 15.19 Causes of splenomegaly.

Gastrointestinal examination	
General	lie patient flat with arms at side wasting, scars, liver flap (asterixis), cock wrists —Hands—clubbing, leuconychia, spider nevi, palmar erythema, Dupuytren's —Head—jaundice, anemia, purpura —Mouth—telangiectasia, pigmentation, ulceration, tongue, hepatic factor (sweet smell) —Supraclavicular node (Virchow's Ⓛ. Troisier's sign.) —Chest wall—gynecomastia, spider nevi, bruising/purpura, muscle wasting
Observe abdomen	—breathe in deeply, cough —areas of fullness, masses, ascites —visible pulsation (aneurysm) —scars, striae —peristalsis —distended veins, direction of flow —hernias —everted umbilicus (ascites)
Palpate abdomen	—ask if tender, watch patient's face, kneel down —gentle palpation in each quadrant, for masses, tenderness —deep palpation —palpate liver from ®iliac fossa, with inspiration, size, border smoothness, tenderness —palpate spleen from ®iliac fossa with inspiration (cf. kidney—cannot get above spleen, dull to percussion, moves with resp, can't ballot). Turn onto ® feel under Ⓛ costal margin —palpate kidneys—bimanually, ballot —palpate for aortic aneurysm
Percussion	—liver, spleen —shifting dullness—center of abdomen to flank, mark point, roll patient to side, back toward umbilicus —fluid thrill—examiner's hand on midline, flick one side, detect on other
Auscultate	—bowel sounds —bruits aorta, hepatic, renal
Hernial orifices	—cough
Genitalla	
PR	
Urinalysis	

Fig. 15.20 A summary of the abdominal examination.

Features on general Inspection in an anemic patient	
Cause	**Features**
iron deficiency*	koilonychia (spoon-shaped nails); painless glossitis; angular stomatitis
hereditary hemorrhagic telangiectasia	visible telangiectasia on face and mouth
Peutz-Jegher's syndrome	pigmented macules around the lips and mouth
megaloblastic anemia*	mild jaundice (lemon-yellow tinge) due to ineffective erythropoiesis; beefy red swollen tongue; angular stomatitis
perncious anemia	usually middle-aged or elderly female; look for features of other autoimmune disease (e.g., vitiligo)

Fig. 15.21 Features on general inspection of a patient with anemia. Asterisks indicate the more common causes.

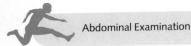

Note racial origin. For example:

- Mediterranean: thalassemia.
- African-American: sickle cell anemia.
- Northern European: hereditary spherocytosis.

Look for causes of blood loss

A systematic survey for a potential source of blood loss should be performed. For example:

- Abdominal scars.
- Gastrointestinal (GI) bleeding: look for abdominal masses; a rectal examination is mandatory.
- Genitourinary source: look for a palpable bladder or kidneys; perform urinalysis.

Look for features of a chronic disease

Look for features of chronic disease such as:

- Infections (e.g., tuberculosis, osteomyelitis, infective endocarditis).
- Connective tissue disease.
- Crohn's disease.
- Malignancy.

Exclude pregnancy

Pregnancy may be associated with folate and iron deficiency.

Perform a thorough abdominal examination

Pathology of the GI tract may cause anemia. For example:

- GI bleeding, malabsorption (e.g., due to celiac disease): iron deficiency anemia.
- Gastrectomy, blind loop syndrome, Crohn's disease: anemia due to folate or vitamin B_{12} deficiency.

In addition an intra-abdominal malignancy may be detected.

Organomegaly is associated with different types of anemia:

- Liver disease is associated with macrocytic anemia.
- Splenomegaly may be responsible for hemolytic anemia.
- A large uterus may be due to pregnancy or be a cause for blood loss.
- Polycystic kidneys may be a cause of chronic renal failure and consequent anemia.

Look for signs of hemolysis

Splenomegaly or mild jaundice may indicate that the underlying cause is hemolysis.

Assess severity of anemia

Try to make an assessment of the functional consequences of the anemia. It is often hard to correlate the degree of pallor with the hemoglobin level. The functional impact of anemia depends upon the underlying condition, the age and fitness of the patient, and the speed of onset. Look for signs of decompensation. For example:

- Hypotension: rapid blood loss may result in hypovolemia and hypotension; postural blood pressure is the most sensitive indicator.
- Tachycardia: this develops early as a means of increasing oxygen delivery to the peripheral tissues in anemia.
- Dyspnea: note the exercise tolerance of a patient (e.g., short of breath at rest or on climbing onto the examination table).
- Heart failure, especially in the elderly.

Acute gastrointestinal bleed

Assess the functional impact

This is a medical emergency. Do not struggle on your own trying to sort this out. It is a team effort, which requires senior support and involvement. If you come across a patient with a significant GI bleed, as a student get help. The initial examination should follow the standard routine of airway, breathing, and circulation (ABCs). When a problem is identified, it must be treated before moving on. It is important to recognize which patients are in danger of exsanguination. The process of assessment and emergency treatment should run in parallel.

Determine the site of bleeding

It is often clear that the bleeding is from the upper or lower GI tract. The vast majority of patients presenting with an acute GI bleed have a lesion at the level of the duodenum or above. Features to suggest an upper GI tract source of bleeding include:

- Hematemesis. Exclude hemoptysis or epistaxis with swallowing and subsequent vomiting of blood.
- Frank blood or "coffee ground" material in the nasogastric (NG) aspirate.
- Absence of a bilious NG aspirate.
- Melena. It is essential to perform a rectal examination. A melena stool indicates bleeding proximal to the right colon and bleeding of usually more than 500 mL in the previous 24 hours. Note

134

that the presence of blood per rectum does not always indicate a lower GI bleed because a very brisk upper GI bleed can result in apparently fresh blood per rectum.

Features of a lower GI bleed include the passage of bright-red blood per rectum (hematochezia). This is not pathognomonic (see above), but if the bleeding is from the upper GI tract, the patient will invariably be profoundly hypovolemic. Common causes of a lower GI bleed are hemorrhoids and diverticular disease.

Perform a detailed abdominal examination

A systematic abdominal examination may provide further clues to the cause. For example:
- Abdominal masses (tumors, diverticular masses, abdominal aortic aneutysm [AAA]).
- Signs of liver disease. GI bleeding is common in liver failure, particularly of an alcoholic etiology.
- Surgical scars. May indicate previous peptic ulcer disease, for example.
- Rectal examination findings. Note stool color. This may indicate the location of the bleeding point as well as the speed of bleeding.

The examination is aimed at assessing the degree of hypovolemia, rate of blood loss, source of bleeding, and urgency of resuscitation. The initial hemoglobin estimate may be misleading, so the requirement for blood transfusion relies upon thorough clinical assessment.

Acute abdominal pain

Acute abdominal pain is one of the most common causes of presentation to an emergency department.

The differential diagnosis is vast, ranging from trivial conditions to life-threatening surgical emergencies. It is important to adopt a systematic approach to the examination. Consider the differential diagnosis throughout the examination (see Fig. 6.3) so that further management strategies

can be instituted efficiently. The main aims of the examination are:
- To establish the cause of pain.
- To assess whether the patient would benefit from admission to hospital.
- To assess whether the patient requires surgical intervention.

General inspection

Before specifically examining the abdomen, look at the patient as a whole. It is helpful to ask the following questions.

Does the patient look unwell?

Patients with acute peritonitis usually look obviously unwell. They are uninterested in their surroundings and lie still so as not to aggravate the pain. Patients with renal colic may also appear distressed but tend to be restless and in obvious pain. Conversely, patients who are laughing, smiling, or eating are most unlikely to have any significant acute surgical disease.

How old is the patient?

Different diseases are more common in different age groups. For example:
- Acute diverticulitis or AAA is much more common with increasing age.
- Acute appendicitis is most common in young children and adolescents but occurs in all age groups.
- Ectopic pregnancy is going to occur only in women of childbearing age.

Which sex is the patient?

In women the differential diagnosis needs to be broadened to include gynecological conditions. The other causes of intra-abdominal pain can occur in either sex, but some have a tendency to be more common in one sex. For example:
- Gallstones are more common in women.
- Peptic ulceration is more common in men.

Specific inspection

Perform a more specific inspection starting at the head and working down to the feet, noting the following.

General appearance

Cachexia may be due to chronic illness or malignancy.

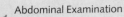
Jaundice

The presence of jaundice should alert the doctor to:
- Gallstones: obstruction of the common bile duct, cholecystitis, pancreatitis.
- Chronic liver disease: associated with gastritis, acute alcoholic hepatitis, and pancreatitis as well as esophageal varices.

Conjunctival pallor

In the context of acute abdominal pain, it may be hard to assess skin coloration as the patient often appears pale, gray, and sweaty. However, conjunctival pallor may suggest the presence of a chronic bleeding lesion. For example:
- Peptic ulcer.
- Colonic tumor with subsequent obstruction or intussusception.

Stigmata of chronic liver disease

See explanation of jaundice above.

Fever

The presence of fever suggests that an active inflammatory process is present.

Left supraclavicular lymphadenopathy

This is suggestive of intra-abdominal malignancy.

Check vital signs

It is essential to check the vital signs as a baseline and to determine the urgency of therapy. Check the following.

Oral temperature

Even in the presence of peritonitis and active infection the patient may not have a fever, especially if in shock. However, the presence of pyrexia indicates that organic pathology is almost invariably present.

Pulse rate

It is unusual to have a tachycardia in the absence of active pathology. However, a very anxious patient may have tachycardia. The sequential recording of pulse rate is an accurate indicator of systemic disturbance if there is a progressive tachycardia. Equally, a completely normal pulse in the presence of severe acute abdominal pathology is unusual. However, beware reliance on the pulse if the patient is on beta-blockers.

Blood pressure

Check supine blood pressure. If the patient is able to cooperate, it is useful to check postural blood pressure. If the patient has shock or hypovolemia, there will be a drop in blood pressure on standing.

Assess fluid status

If the jugular venous waveform is easily visible, the jugular venous pressure provides a useful marker of fluid status.

Abdominal examination
Inspection

Inspect the abdomen noting:
- Visible peristalsis: suggestive of obstruction.
- Abdominal distension: may be due to obstruction.
- Rigidity: a tense, boardlike abdomen occurs in the presence of peritonitis.
- Any skin discoloration: pancreatitis may be associated with a bluish discoloration in the flank due to extravasation of bloodstained pancreatic fluid into the retroperitoneum.
- Obvious hernias.
- Abdominal scars: their presence raises the possibility of obstruction due to adhesions.
- Obvious organomegaly: for example, massive polycystic kidneys may cause bulging in the flank. Bleeding into a cyst may be the cause for the pain.

Note the site of the pain

Ask the patient to show you exactly where the pain is on the abdomen. The location of the pain is the key to the underlying cause (see Fig. 6.2).

Examine the abdomen in detail

Perform a detailed abdominal examination as described at the start of this chapter. In particular, note:
- Presence or absence of signs of peritonitis.
- Presence of any abdominal masses.
- Location of the tenderness.

Signs of peritonitis

The presence of unexplained peritonitis is an indication for surgical intervention. The features of peritonitis are:
- Signs of shock (tachycardia, hypotension, which becomes progressive on serial observation; Fig. 15.22).
- Tenderness.
- Guarding (a sign of severe tenderness).

Fig. 15.22 This figure shows the four stages of shock. Note how much blood you have to lose before your blood pressure drops.

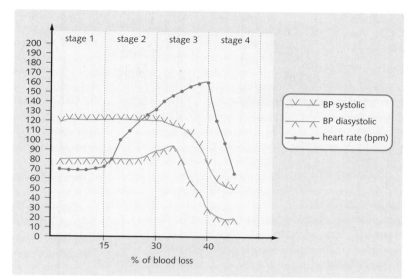

Causes of a right iliac fossa mass	
Causes	**Features**
appendix mass	preceding history of central abdominal pain moving to the right iliac fossa; anorexia; tender mass; persistent fever and tachycardia; tender per rectum (PR)
carcinoma of the cecum	firm distinct mass; often nonmobile; usually nontender; patient does not look acutely unwell
tuberculosis	more common in patients from the Indian subcontinent or Africa
Crohn's disease	patient may appear hypovolemic owing to diarrhea; oral aphthous ulcers; skin tags; mass usually mobile and of rubbery consistency; tender mass
psoas abscess	ill-defined mass; lumbar tenderness
iliac lymph nodes	
iliac artery aneurysm	

Fig. 15.23 Causes of a right iliac fossa mass.

- Rebound tenderness. This is a useful discriminatory sign since many anxious patients have involuntary guarding upon palpation, but do not expect tenderness on withdrawal of the palpating hand. The tenderness may be distant to the site of palpation. Watch the patient's face for signs of rebound tenderness.
- Localized pain distant to the site of palpation.
- Absent bowel sounds.

Presence of an abdominal mass

Examination of palpable liver, spleen, and kidney is discussed on pp. 126–127. In the context of acute abdominal pain, a mass in the right or left iliac fossa is most relevant.

Mass in the right iliac fossa

The most common causes are an appendix mass or carcinoma of the cecum. The differential diagnosis is shown in Fig. 15.23.

Mass in the left iliac fossa

The same diseases as shown in Fig 15.23 may cause a left iliac fossa mass, except for carcinoma of the cecum, Crohn's disease, and tuberculosis. Diverticulitis is common and may cause a mass.

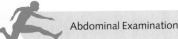

Carcinoma of the colon usually presents with weight loss or a change in bowel habit, but occasionally presents as a left iliac fossa mass, especially if it is causing obstruction.

Location of the pain
Generalized
Generalized abdominal pain is likely to be due to generalized peritonitis. The history is central to the diagnosis.

Epigastric
The most common causes of epigastric pain are:
- Peptic ulcer.
- A biliary cause (biliary colic or cholecystitis).
- Pancreatitis.

Peptic ulcer usually produces no signs unless perforation has occurred, though pyloric stenosis may result in visible peristalsis.

Biliary pain is more common in the right upper quadrant. Often there are no abdominal signs, though there is commonly tenderness in the right upper quadrant upon inspiration.

Pancreatitis often produces surprisingly few abdominal signs for the degree of shock.

The conditions that cause abdominal pain, shock, and a soft abdomen are:
- Pancreatitis.
- Bowel infarction.
- Dissection of an AAA.
- Referred pain from a myocardial infarction.

Flank pain
The main causes of flank pain are:
- Renal colic.
- Pyelonephritis.
- Musculoskeletal pain.

Right iliac fossa pain
The most important cause of right iliac fossa pain is acute appendicitis. However, the differential diagnosis is wide. Other causes include:
- Gastroenteritis.
- Mesenteric adenitis.
- Ruptured ovarian cyst.
- Acute salpingitis.
- Perforated peptic ulcer.
- Acute cholecystitis.

- Crohn's disease.
- Acute diverticulitis (rarely on the right).
- Renal colic.
- Ectopic pregnancy.

Medical conditions
It is important to remember that medical conditions may present with acute abdominal pain, so a detailed systemic examination is essential. In particular, examine:
- The cardiovascular system. Inferior myocardial infarction or angina occasionally presents with predominantly upper abdominal pain.
- The respiratory system. Pneumonia (especially with lower lobar disease) may cause right or left upper quadrant pain. Look for signs of consolidation.
- Diabetic ketoacidosis.

Chronic renal failure

Patients with chronic renal failure often have specific problems, which should always be considered during an assessment. For dialysis patients, consider the following points.

Assess dialysis access
Hemodialysis
Note the presence of the arteriovenous fistula (AVF), its site (e.g., radial, brachial), and the palpable thrill. Look for access sites used and other possible access sites, include Gore-Tex graft, shunts, or central venous catheters.

Look specifically for signs of infection (especially with venous catheters).

Peritoneal dialysis
Look at the exit site of the peritoneal dialysis catheter for evidence of tunnel infection or exit site infection. If the patient has reported abdominal symptoms, it is important to inspect the dialysis fluid for turbidity, blood, or cloudiness suggestive of peritonitis.

Assess fluid balance
Fluid overload is a common problem in anuric patients.

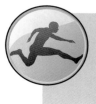

Measure the patient's weight at every visit. This is the most sensitive guide to changes in fluid balance on a day-to-day basis.

Do not forget the original disease causing the renal failure!

Look for other signs of fluid overload such as:
- Raised JVP.
- Peripheral edema: if the patient has a normal plasma albumin, peripheral edema usually indicates a fluid overload of approximately 3 kg.
- Uncontrolled hypertension.
- Pulmonary edema: often a combination of fluid overload and cardiac failure.

Some patients develop symptoms such as lightheadedness, fainting, or malaise toward the end of dialysis. Look for signs of dehydration such as:
- Dry mucous membranes.
- Postural hypotension.

Check lying and standing blood pressure

Most dialysis patients have hypertension, and pristine blood pressure control is central to reducing long-term morbidity from cardiac disease. Postural blood pressure assessment is useful for determining fluid balance. Erythropoietin therapy may exacerbate hypertension.

Look for activity of underlying disease

It is important to remember the underlying cause of renal failure as this may cause special problems in management. For example:
- The diabetic patient has a particularly high risk of cardiovascular disease.
- A patient with a vasculitic illness may develop recurrent vasculitis with extrarenal complications (e.g., pulmonary hemorrhage).
- Amyloidosis may progress causing systemic complications.

Perform a full systemic examination

Renal failure is a multisystem disease, and a full assessment is essential.

Palpable kidneys

It is unusual to be able to palpate normal kidneys in any but very lean patients. If a kidney is palpable, it is necessary to:
- Identify the mass as a kidney.
- Consider the underlying cause.

Identify the mass as a kidney

The right kidney is often palpable in a thin subject; the left is palpable less often. Features of an enlarged palpable kidney include:
- Location in the flank (paracolic gutter).
- It is usually possible to palpate only the lower pole.
- Downward movement on inspiration (the spleen tends to move toward the right iliac fossa).
- Usually resonant to percussion (see spleen or liver, p. 126; it is overlaid by the colon).
- It can be balloted (almost a pathognomonic sign).
- It may be possible to "get above" the mass (compare directly with the liver or spleen).

A palpable kidney is rarely confused with any other organ, but it should be clearly differentiated from the spleen on the left and the liver on the right (Fig. 15.24).

Define the characteristics of the kidney

Once the organ has been identified as the kidney, define the size, consistency, and shape. Listen over the organ for a bruit, which may be present if there is renal artery stenosis or a tumor.

Consider etiology
Bilateral palpable kidneys

The most common causes of bilaterally palpable kidneys are:

139

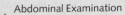
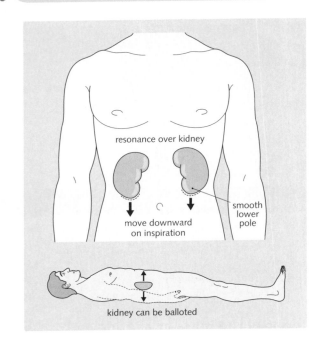

resonance over kidney

move downward on inspiration

smooth lower pole

kidney can be balloted

Fig. 15.24 Features of a palpable kidney.

- Bilateral hydronephrosis.
- Amyloidosis. The patient may have a typical facies, hepatosplenomegaly, peripheral neuropathy, or obvious underlying inflammatory disease (e.g., rheumatoid arthritis, chronic osteomyelitis).

Other causes are shown in Fig. 15.25.

Unilateral palpable kidney
The most common causes are similar, but in order of frequency include:
1. Polycystic kidneys.
2. Renal cell carcinoma.
3. Hydronephrosis.
4. Hypertrophy of a single functioning kidney (kidney only just palpable).

- Polycystic kidneys (the most common cause). The kidneys may be massive. Most other causes result in smooth hemiovoid masses, but occasionally individual cysts may be palpable. Look for an associated polycystic liver, signs of uremia, or an arteriovenous fistula.

 Do not forget to check the urinalysis. Transplanted kidneys are normally placed in the right iliac fossa.

Causes of enlarged kidneys, single or bilateral	
Causes	**Features**
polycystic kidneys	usually bilateral; large cysts may be individually detected; check blood pressure; note uremic complications; may detect hepatomegaly
hydronephrosis	unilateral or bilateral; may be tender if acute; check prostate and palpable bladder
malignancy Wilms' tumor (child) renal cell carcinoma (hypernephroma)	look for systemic features of malignancy
miscellaneous pyonephrosis single cyst amyloid	 tender usually incidental finding rare; look for underlying disease

Fig. 15.25 Causes of single or bilaterally enlarged kidneys.

16. Obstetric and Gynecological Examination

Overview

Taking an obstetrics or gynecology history does not differ from the standard history format outlined in Chapter 2. However, there are some specialist questions that need to asked. It is important to remember that this is a sensitive area for many women who many not feel comfortable discussing certain topics with medical students, especially male medical students.

The gynecological history

This should include:

Menstrual history

- Ask about the menarche and, if appropriate, the menopause.
- When was the first day of the last menstrual cycle?
- The pattern of bleeding and the length of time between cycles. It is important to remember that the menstrual cycle is from the first day of bleeding to the next first day of bleeding. Try to establish the pattern of bleeding. How many days does this last, what kind of protection is used, how often does it need to be changed, does the woman ever flood through her protection, and does she ever pass clots?
- Ask the patient about menstrual pain. For example, does the pain begin before menstruation, is it relieved by menstruation, or is menstruation itself painful? Try to determine the severity of pain and its functional impact on the woman's life. What analgesics does she use and for how long? Does she have any other associated cyclical symptoms?

Try and remember at all times what is happening to the patient's hormone level throughout the normal menstrual cycle (Fig. 16.1).

Contraception and sexual history

A contraceptive history should be taken. This should include which methods have been tried and how suitable the women considered them to be.

If appropriate, you may need to ask about the woman's sexual history. Is she sexually active? Do not make assumptions about her sexuality or sexual orientation. This is a very sensitive area, and great care should be taken in asking about sexual history. It is often a good idea to leave this topic until the end of the interview when you have had the most amount of time to build up a rapport. Sexual history should include the number of partners that she has had over the past year and the sex of the partners. Ask how often she has had intercourse and, if appropriate, whether or not she had dyspareunia. You should also ask if she has had any sexually transmitted diseases.

Pap smear tests

You should also ask when the patient's last pap smear test was. Has she been attending a clinic and has she had any abnormal pap smears? What treatment did she require for these?

Vaginal discharge and continence

Symptoms of any vaginal discharge should be recorded. When does it occur (when during the cycle, postcoital or postmenopausal), how much is there and its nature (consistency, color, smell), and is there any blood?

Ask about urinary abnormalities (e.g., frequency, nocturia, dysuria). Are there any symptoms of stress incontinence (usually a consequence of lax pelvic musculature following childbirth) or urge incontinence (usually due to detrusor instability)?

The obstetric history

Pregnancy is usually a happy time for people, but there may also be a lot of anxiety, especially if previous pregnancies have been lost. You should find out about the current pregnancy first.

Ask about the last menstrual period, and then calculate her expected due date.

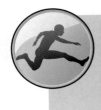

A favorite examination question involves working out a woman's date for delivery using the gestational calendar. Find one and practice with it.

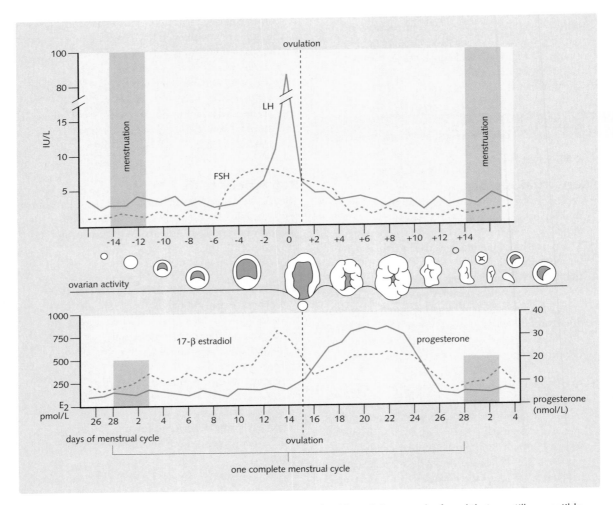

Fig. 16.1 Hormone levels in the normal menstrual cycle. Considerable variations can be found that are still compatible with normal menstrual function.

Was there any difficulty in getting pregnant? Ask whether she has had any of the symptoms of pregnancy, such as early morning sickness. You may ask about any cravings. Has the mother felt any fetal activity yet?

Previous obstetric history

- How many times has she been pregnant, and how many children does she have? This is a delicate way of starting to find out about miscarriages and abortions.
- Are all of the children to one father? If not, clarify the paternities.
- When the children were born, what was their gestation? Did any of them have to go to a special care baby unit?
- Have there been any fetal abnormalities or any postnatal complications?
- During her previous pregnancies did she have any medical problems, such as pre-eclampsia or diabetes?
- Were her previous labors difficult? What did she use for analgesia? Was it satisfactory?
- Did she require instrumental deliveries or cesarean sections?
- Has she had any postnatal psychological problems, such as postpartum depression?

You should also take a gynecological history as outlined above.

When asking about medications, find out whether or not she is taking folic acid.

It is important to take a family and a social history. Particular attention should be paid to any inherited diseases that run in the family, such as cystic fibrosis. It is also useful to know if there is a history of twins in the family. Ask the mother about her marital status. Ask if she is employed and how long she intends to work while pregnant. Is the home suitable for children, or will she need to be rehoused? Does she still drink alcohol? If so, how much? Does she smoke? Again, if so, how much? The mother should be encouraged to stop or at least cut down smoking and drinking. This is also a good opportunity to find out if the woman is considering breastfeeding.

When dealing with pregnant mothers, remember that pregnancy is not a disease state. Most pregnancies are uncomplicated and do not require medical interventions. At times we can become biased in our views of pregnancy because we see and remember the problematic patients. You need to decide for yourself what you feel about medical interventions in pregnancy and what an appropriate level of medical involvement is.

17. Surgical Examination

Overview

This chapter details how to examine some surgical pathologies. You need to be proficient at many different examinations. This chapter should be used in conjunction with hands-on bedside teaching.

Lumps in the groin

This method covers all of the salient special tests that you will be expected to perform to evaluate a lump in the groin.

First, expose the patient's abdomen. The standard teaching is nipples to knees, but umbilicus to knees will normally suffice.

- Look at the patient lying down.
- Can you see any obvious swelling? Where is it? Is it superior or inferior to the inguinal ligament, or is it in the scrotum? What color is it? Is it erythematous?
- Are there any scars from previous surgery?
- If nothing can be seen, then ask the patient to stand. Can you see anything now?

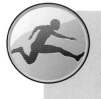 We have two of most things for easy comparison. Don't forget to check for contralateral pathology in the heat of the moment.

Next, define the swelling. Lumps have three dimensions: measure the length, breadth, and depth. There is likely to be a measuring tape located at the bedside, so use it. Now that you have its size, define its shape.

- Is the lump fluctuant? Can you transilluminate it? When you feel it, does it extend beyond the obvious skin markings?
- Test the lump for a cough impulse. Place your hand over the swelling and ask the patient to cough. Does the swelling get worse?

Ask patients to reduce the swelling themselves. Put pressure over the deep inguinal ring (halfway between the pubic tubercle and the anterior superior iliac spine), and ask the patient to cough. If a swelling appears medial to the pressure, it is a direct hernia. Release the pressure, and ask the patient to cough again. If the hernia appears now, it is an indirect hernia (Fig. 17.1).

Next check the other side for any similar defects.

Differential diagnosis of groin swellings
Above the inguinal ligament
- Sebaceous cyst, lipoma.
- Direct/indirect inguinal hernia.
- Imperfectly descended testis.

Below the inguinal ligament
- Sebaceous cyst, lipoma, lymph nodes.
- Femoral hernia.
- Saphena varix (dilatation of the saphenous vein at the confluence with the femoral vein).
- Femoral aneurysm (expansile pulsation, bruit, not compressible with no cough impulse).
- Imperfectly descended testis.
- Psoas abscess (rare).

Alternatively, think of the mass in terms of structure as in Fig. 17.2.

Scrotal swellings

Examination
Observe the swelling from the anterior and posterior aspects of the scrotum. Define its size and shape, and note the skin color.

Gently palpate the swelling. This is best achieved by rolling the testes between the thumb and finger. Find and feel the epididymis and feel the spermatic cord.

Try to assess the swelling. What is its size, shape, and fluctuance? Does it transilluminate? There ought to be a light at the bedside of these patients. Can the upper edge of the mass be felt (e.g., can you get above it)? Is it separate from the testes?

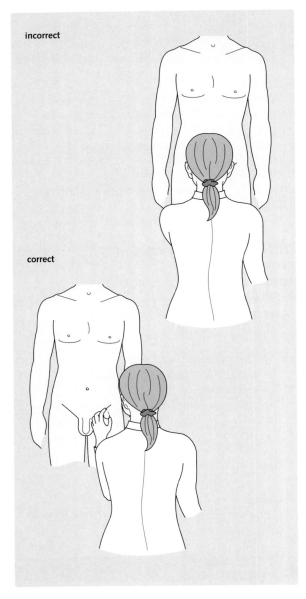

incorrect

correct

Fig. 17.1 Examination of a hernia. If examining a swelling, stand at the patient's side.

Differential diagnoses of lumps in the grain	
hernias	inguinal/femoral
vascular	saphena varix/femoral aneurysm
lymph nodes	lymphadenopathy (infection/neoplasm/lymphoma)
muscles	psoas abscess
testicular	ectopic testes
skin/subcutaneous	lipoma/sebaceous cyst

Fig. 17.2 Differential diagnoses of lumps in the groin.

Peripheral vascular disease

Patients with peripheral vascular disease are challenging to examine. They have multiple medical problems, all of which need to be investigated. This is an approach to examining their limbs.

Expose both legs completely, while preserving the patient's dignity. This includes taking off the socks. If a dressing is in place, it should be taken down and the underlying wound inspected. You should have a nurse to help you if this needs to be done.

Inspect both legs and feet for:
- The color of the skin. Is it white, red, or black? Each is associated with differing degrees of vascular insufficiency.
- Trophic changes. For example, is the skin smooth and shiny? Is there loss of hair (note where this occurs) or wasting of subcutaneous tissue? Careful note should be made of any ulcers. All ulcers should be examined. Please see p. 149 for how to do this.
- Look specifically at the pressure points in the limb for ulcers. Pay special attention to the lateral aspect of the foot, the head of the 1st metatarsophalangeal, the heel, and malleoli.
- Finally, inspect the tips of the toes and between the toes. Patients are often immobile and unable to care for their feet. A small lesion here can rapidly progress.

Palpation of both legs:
- Feel both legs for a difference in temperature. Note the level of any temperature change.

Your differential should run along these lines:
- Cystic, testicular, and not usually tender: hydrocele (Fig. 17.3A).
- Cystic, separate, and not usually tender: epididymal cyst (Fig. 17.3B).
- Solid and testicular: tumor, orchitis (very tender), granuloma, gumma (Fig. 17.3C).
- Solid, separate, and usually tender: chronic epididymitis (Fig. 17.3D).

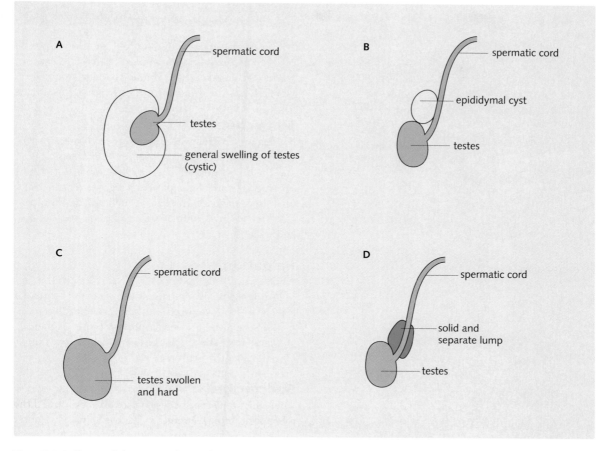

Fig. 17.3 Differential diagnoses of scrotal swellings.

- Count the capillary refill time in both feet or stumps (press on the nailbed for 5 seconds and count; the capillary refill should be less than 2 seconds).
- Feel for all pulses in the legs (femoral, popliteal, dorsalis pedis, and posterior tibial). Classify the pulse as normal, diminished, or absent. Figure 17.4 shows the arterial tree of the lower limb.

Auscultate and listen along the major vessels for arterial bruits.

Special tests

Elevate the leg to 15° and look for venous guttering. Keep elevating the leg until it becomes white (ischemic) and note the angle. This is known as Buerger's angle and is normally >90°. From this elevated position lower the leg over the side of the bed and look for reactive hyperemia (this is Buerger's test).

There is often a Doppler ultrasound probe around (especially in examinations). This is used to measure the ankle/brachial pressure index. Take a blood pressure in the ankle with the Doppler probe and a brachial blood pressure with the Doppler probe. Divide the ankle pressure by the brachial pressure to give a ratio (Fig. 17.5).

You should also examine the patient's cardiovascular system for other signs of arterial disease and an aortic aneurysm.

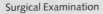

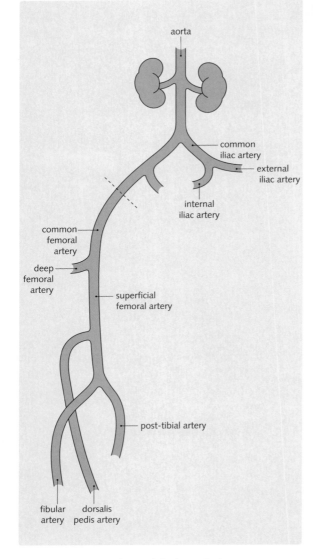

Fig. 17.4 The arterial tree of the lower limb.

ABPI	Significance
1–1.2	Normal
0.8	Claudication pain
0.4	Rest pain
<0.4	Ulceration and gangrene

Fig. 17.5 Ankle/brachial pressure index (ABPI).

Varicose veins

Varicose veins are a common problem. They are often found in outpatient clinics and day surgery wards. When asked to examine a patient's varicose veins, follow the usual pattern.

Inspection

Maintaining patient modesty, expose both legs with the patient standing up. Observe the patient's legs and the distribution of the varicose veins. Note the nutritional state of the patient's legs (especially the area superior to the medial malleolus). You should also look for any eczematous changes, pigmentation, and varicose ulcers.

Palpation

Palpate and compare both legs. Is there a difference in temperature? Is the patient tender over the medial aspect of the lower leg? You should specifically palpate the ankle for dermatoliposclerosis. Is there ankle edema? These signs give an indication of the chronicity of the problem.

Specific tests

There are some special tests that you should perform when examining someone's varicose veins.

Feel the saphenofemoral junction (4 cm inferior and lateral to the pubic tubercule—remember Fig. 17.1). Is there a swelling here? If so, it is likely to be a saphena varix. With your fingers on the saphenofemoral junction ask the patient to cough. If you feel an impulse, it is suggestive of venous incompetence. Last, perform the percussion test. Tap the top of the vein and feel below for an impulse; if one is present, it is suggestive of superficial venous incompetence.

You should now ask the patient to lie down and elevate the leg to empty the veins. Place two fingers on the saphenofemoral junction and ask the patient to stand. As you are doing this, carefully observe the leg. If the veins rapidly fill, then the lower leg perforators are incompetent. Now release your fingers. If there is rapid filling of the leg, the patient has an incompetent saphenofemoral valve.

To conclude your examination, you should examine the abdomen for any masses. If you are suspicious of an obstruction, a per rectum exam should be done. It is rare to do this in practice.

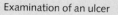

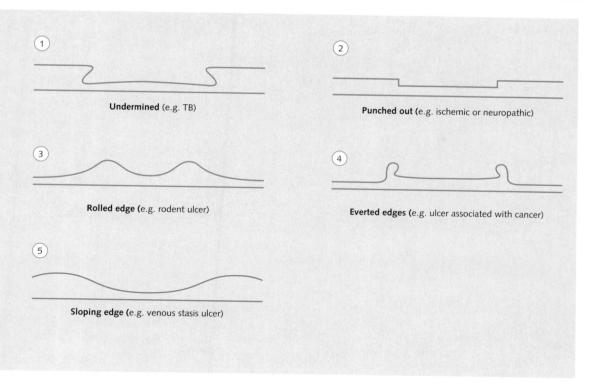

Fig. 17.6 Classification of an ulcer.

Examination of an ulcer

An ulcer is a break in the continuity of an epithelial surface. Ulcers are associated with a number of conditions, some of which have been discussed above. At some point in your career someone will present you with an ulcer and ask your opinion about it. It helps to have a system to help describe it.

Inspection

Remove all of the dressing and gently clean off any topical applications. Expose the whole ulcer completely. Inspect the ulcer, noting:

- Its position, size, and shape.
- The base (color, penetration of underlying structures such as tendon/bone).
- Any discharge from the ulcer (blood, pus, or serous fluid).
- Measure the depth of the ulcer in millimeters.
- Inspect the edge (Fig. 17.6).
- Feel the surrounding tissues for any tenderness or temperature changes.
- Note the nutrition of surrounding tissue, and check for regional lymph nodes.
- You should also make an assessment of the neurovascular supply to the area (e.g., sensation and muscle power).

18. Neurological Examination

Examination routine

The neurological examination is often considered to be the most difficult part of the examination by students and is most commonly omitted or performed poorly. In a full routine assessment, it is essential to perform at least a basic neurological assessment. This need not take more than a few minutes but provides essential information.

More than in any other system, it is vital to be systematic, objective, and methodical and to be aware of the pathological significance of any elicited sign. It is essential to record exactly what has been assessed rather than using meaningless phrases (e.g., "CNS—tick"). Interpretation of neurological conditions often relies on changes of neurological signs with time, highlighting the need to ensure accuracy in writing up the medical record.

The complete neurological examination includes:
- Mental status (see Chapter 9).
- Cranial nerves.
- Motor function.
- Sensory function.
- Reflexes.
- Cerebellar function.

Cranial nerves

It is important to understand the basic anatomy and function of the individual cranial nerves in interpreting physical findings. Function, anatomy, examination routine, and interpretation of the physical signs are considered below for each cranial nerve.

Olfactory nerve (cranial nerve I)
Function
The olfactory nerve is a sensory nerve conveying the sense of smell.

Anatomy
Nerve fibers pass from sensory receptors in the nasal cavity through the cribriform plate to the olfactory bulb, where they synapse, and then pass toward the anterior perforated substance.

Examination
Ask patients whether they have noticed any change in their sense of smell. Test smell in each nostril separately using a sniff test. Use common, easily recognizable, nonirritant substances (e.g., vanilla, orange, coffee).

Interpretation
It is relatively unusual to detect lesions of the olfactory nerve on physical examination. Formal testing is rarely needed unless a lesion of the anterior cranial fossa is suspected. If a lesion is detected, note the following:
- Anosmia is usually due to nasal rather than neurological disease.
- The olfactory nerve is vulnerable as it passes through the cribriform plate, especially if there is a head injury. Also consider frontal lobe tumors and meningitis (infective or neoplastic).

Optic nerve (cranial nerve II)
Function
The optic nerve is a sensory nerve conveying the sense of vision from the retina.

Anatomy
The optic nerve leaves the eye via the optic foramen, partially decussates at the optic chiasm, and synapses at the lateral geniculate nucleus. Secondary fibers pass to the occipital cortex via the optic radiation (see "Interpretation" below).

Examination
Visual acuity Assess distant and near vision formally with Snellen and Jaeger charts, allowing patients to wear their glasses, or crudely at the bedside (e.g., count fingers from 2 meters or read newsprint) for each eye.

Visual fields Test by confrontation. Sit opposite the patient so that you are approximately 1 meter apart at the same level. Both of you should then cover one eye, and you bring a test object (traditionally a white hatpin) into the field of vision from each quadrant midway between yourself and the patient. The patient states when he or she first sees the object, and you can then compare the patient's visual field directly with yours.

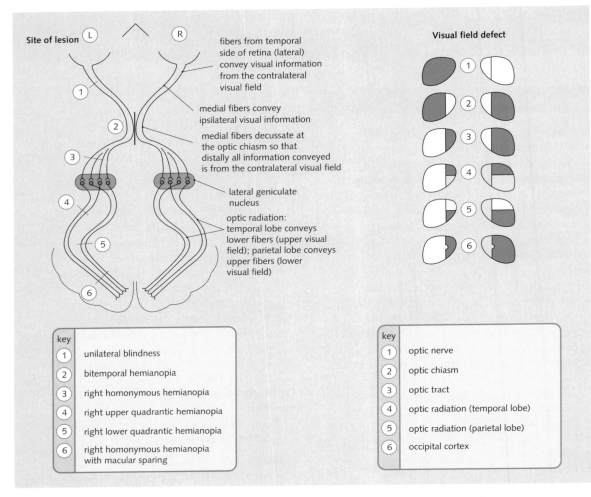

Fig. 18.1 The visual pathway. Lesions at different parts of the pathway produce characteristic field defects.

Pupillary reflexes. These are discussed under oculomotor nerve (see p. 153).

Fundoscopy. See Chapter 23 for details.

Interpretations

Visual field defects should be correlated with the anatomical site of the lesion. It is helpful to understand the visual pathway (Fig. 18.1).

Oculomotor, trochlear, and abducens nerves (cranial nerves III, IV, VI)

Function

The oculomotor, trochlear, and abducens nerves are considered together as they supply the extraocular muscles (Fig. 18.2). The oculomotor nerve also supplies the levator palpebrae superioris, which opens the upper eyelid. In addition, it also has parasympathetic fibers supplying the sphincter pupillae (which constricts the pupil) and the ciliary muscle of the lens.

Anatomy

The oculomotor nucleus lies in the midbrain. It passes close to the posterior communicating artery before entering the lateral wall of the cavernous sinus on the way to the orbit.

The trochlear nucleus lies lower in the midbrain. Fibers pass dorsally, decussate, pass around the midbrain, and enter the lateral wall of the cavernous sinus.

The abducens nerve originates close to the facial nerve in the pons, emerges in the cerebellopontine

Fig. 18.2 Nerve supply and movement produced by the extraocular muscles.

Nerve supply and movement produced by the extraocular muscles		
Nerve	**Muscle**	**Movement**
oculomotor	medial rectus	adduction
	inferior rectus	inferior movement (especially when eye abducted)
	superior rectus	superior movement
	inferior oblique	superior movement (especially when eye adducted)
trochlear	superior oblique	inferior movement (especially when eye adducted)
abducens	lateral rectus	abduction

Causes of ptosis	
Cause	**Examples**
third nerve palsy complete ptosis, associated with widely dilated pupil, and eye paralyzed with outward and downward deviation	posterior communicating artery aneurysm "coning" of the temporal lobe mononeuritis multiplex (e.g., due to diabetes mellitus, vasculitis) midbrain lesion
Horner's syndrome loss of sympathetic supply to eye, partial ptosis, pupillary constriction, enophthalmos and decreased sweating on affected side	brain lesion (e.g., CVA lateral medullary syndrome) cervical cord lesion (e.g., syringomyelia) T1 root lesion (e.g., apical lung cancer, cervical rib) sympathetic chain lesion (e.g., neoplasia)
neuromuscular disease	myasthenia gravis botulism
myogenic	senile degenerative changes dystrophia myotonica

Fig. 18.3 Causes of ptosis. CVA, cerebrovascular accident.

angle, and has a very long intracranial course, passing over the petrous temporal bone on the way to the cavernous sinus.

Examination

Inspection   Look at the eyelids for ptosis and symmetry.

Pupils   Look at pupil size and symmetry. Test the pupillary reflex by shining light on the pupil from the side, looking at both the direct and consensual response.

Ocular movements   Observe the patient following a target up, down, to either side, and for convergence. Note diplopia or nystagmus.

Interpretation

When interpreting physical signs, note the following:

- Ptosis (Fig. 18.3).
- Abnormal pupillary reflexes. The afferent limb is from the optic nerve, the efferent pathway is via the oculomotor nerve. An intact consensual reflex with an absent direct reflex implies a lesion of the IIIrd nerve. Conversely, pupil constriction only when light is shone into the opposite eye implies a sensory deficit.
- Holmes–Adie pupil. This is common in normal women. The pupil is large with an absent light reflex and delayed accommodation reflex, which is sustained. It is often associated with absent ankle reflexes.

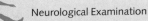

- Nystagmus. This may be due to visual disturbances or lesions of the labyrinth, cerebellum, brainstem, or central vestibular connections. See Nystagmus section, below.
- VIth nerve palsy (loss of eye abduction). This is often a false localizing sign. The VIth nerve has a very long intracranial course and is vulnerable to compression as it passes over the petrous temporal bone. Any pathology causing raised intracranial pressure may result in a VIth nerve palsy.
- VIth nerve lesions may be due to a lesion in the pons or cerebellopontine angle. This often occurs in association with a VIIth (or VIIIth) nerve palsy and may result in contralateral pyramidal tract signs.
- IVth nerve palsy. This rarely occurs in isolation. Orbital trauma often damages the tendon, causing muscular weakness.

Nystagmus

Nystagmus is caused by posterior fossa disease or ear pathology.

First, in which eye is the nystagmus most obvious? Second, is the nystagmus greater when looking to the affected side (e.g., present in the right eye and worse when looking right)? This is the most common situation. Nystagmus is caused by:

- Contralateral vestibular lesion (associated with vertigo and deafness).
- Multiple sclerosis.
- Middle ear surgery.
- Ménière's disease.
- Ipsilateral cerebellar lesion (associated with other cerebellar signs).
- Neoplasia.
- Cerebrovascular accident (CVA).
- Ipsilateral brainstem lesion. These can be infective, vascular (the most likely), neoplastic, or demyelinating in origin.

If the patient has vertical nystagmus, this implies a central lesion. If it is down gaze, consider pathologies around the foramen magnum. If it is up gaze, the lesion will be around the superior colliculus.

Sixth nerve palsy is commonly a false localizing sign and results from raised intracranial pressure.

Trigeminal nerve (cranial nerve V)
Function
The trigeminal nerve conveys sensory and motor nerve fibers. The main functions are:
- Sensory: somatic sensation to the face.
- Motor: muscles of mastication (masseters, temporalis, pterygoids).

Anatomy
The trigeminal nerve is split into the following three divisions (Fig. 18.4):
- Ophthalmic.
- Maxillary.
- Mandibular.

The trigeminal ganglion lies near the pons. The nerve fibers pass near the medial lemniscus to the thalamus.

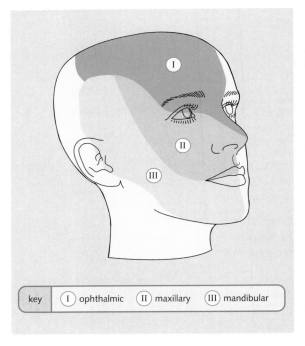

key   (I) ophthalmic   (II) maxillary   (III) mandibular

Fig. 18.4 Dermatomes of the three divisions of the trigeminal nerve.

Examination

Sensory Test modalities of sensation over the three distributions of the nerve (e.g., forehead, cheeks, chin) bilaterally.

Corneal reflex Lightly touch the cornea with cotton wool, approaching from the side, and observe a brisk contraction of orbicularis oris (blinking).

Motor Inspect for wasting of temporalis and masseter. Test jaw opening against resistance (unilateral pterygoid weakness will cause the jaw to deviate to the side of the weakness).

Jaw jerk This is often difficult to interpret.

Interpretation

When examining the Vth nerve, note the following points:

- An absent corneal reflex may be the first sign of ophthalmic herpes. Lesions of the Vth and VIIth nerves can be distinguished by comparing the contralateral responses. The afferent limb is from the Vth nerve; the efferent limb is provided by the facial nerve and is usually bilateral.
- Central lesions are often associated with other localizing signs (e.g., first division in association with IIIrd, IVth, and VIth nerve in the cavernous sinus; cerebellopontine angle lesions).
- Sensory lesions are much more common than motor lesions.

Facial nerve (cranial nerve VII)
Function
The facial nerve is primarily a motor nerve but conveys fibers of three different modalities:

- Motor: to muscles of facial expression.
- Parasympathetic: to lacrimal, submaxillary, and sublingual glands.
- Sensory: taste for the anterior two-thirds of the tongue and sensation to an insignificant part of the external ear.

Anatomy
The motor nucleus lies in the pons close to the VIth nerve. It emerges in the cerebellopontine angle and enters the internal auditory meatus with the VIIIth nerve, giving off the nerve to stapedius and chorda tympani (taste) before emerging through the stylomastoid foramen and passing peripherally through the parotid gland, giving off various branches.

Examination

Inspection Inspect the face for:

- Asymmetry (e.g., loss of nasolabial fold, drooping and dribbling from corner of mouth, weak smile).
- Facial expression.
- Involuntary movements.

Muscle strength Examine the individual muscles. The lower face may be assessed by smiling, whistling, pursing lips; the upper face by closure of eyes, elevation of eyebrows, frowning.

Taste Taste is rarely formally tested.

Interpretation
By far the most important component of the facial nerve is motor. Upper motor neuron (UMN) lesions often result in relative preservation of movements of the upper face due to crossed innervation (Fig. 18.5). In addition, emotional expression may be preserved. Lower motor neuron (LMN) VIIth nerve lesions do not spare the muscles around the eyes. The site of the lesion can often be localized:

- Pons: for example, lesion due to a CVA; associated with VIth nerve lesion and contralateral pyramidal tract signs.
- Cerebellopontine angle: for example, lesion due to an acoustic neuroma; associated with lesions of the VIth, VIIth, and VIIIth nerves as well as cerebellar ataxia.
- Facial canal: for example, lesion due to Bell's palsy, herpes zoster; associated with loss of taste and hyperacusis as well as muscles of facial expression.
- Parotid gland: for example, lesion due to sarcoidosis, parotid tumor; individual facial muscles may be affected.

Vestibulocochlear nerve (cranial nerve VIII)
Function
The vestibulocochlear nerve is a sensory nerve. It has two primary functions:

- Auditory: sense of hearing.
- Labyrinthine: sense of balance.

Anatomy
Auditory Sensory fibers from the cochlea enter the cerebellopontine angle in association with the facial nerve, synapse in the lower pons, and ascend in the lateral lemnisci.

Vestibular Fibers pass with the auditory division, but synapse in the vestibular nucleus in the medulla,

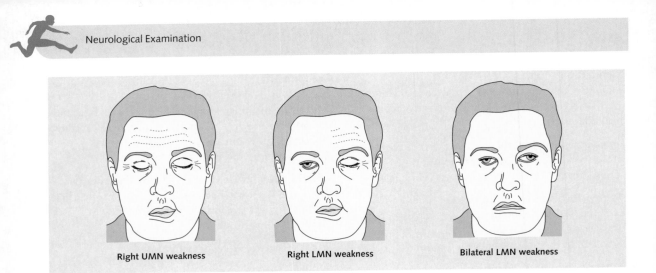

Right UMN weakness   Right LMN weakness   Bilateral LMN weakness

Fig. 18.5 Facial weakness. Patients are asked to close their eyes and purse their lips. Note the failed eye closure in lower motor neuron (LMN) lesions and the nasolabial fold with drooping mouth in both upper motor neuron (UMN) and LMN lesions.

from which there are connections to the cerebellum, extraocular muscles, and higher centers.

Examination

Auditory   Crude assessment can be made for each ear (e.g., "Can hear whispered voice"). If a defect is found, conductive or sensory deficits may be identified using tuning fork tests (Fig. 18.6) as follows:

- Rinne's test: using a 256 Hz tuning fork, compare subjective loudness when it is presented close to the external auditory meatus and when the base is applied to the mastoid. A positive test (normal) occurs if the former appears louder.
- Weber's test: apply the base of the tuning fork to the middle of the forehead and ask the patient whether he or she hears the sound in the midline or to one side. The test is abnormal if the sound is lateralized.

Vestibular   This function is not routinely tested. Positional nystagmus can be observed by holding the patient's head over the end of the examination table and then fully extending and turning it with the eyes open. This test is called Hallpike's maneuver (Fig. 18.7).

Interpretation

If hearing loss is identified, try to identify the underlying cause. Note that:

- Tuning fork tests are useful for identifying the hearing deficit as primarily conductive or sensory in origin (Fig. 18.8).

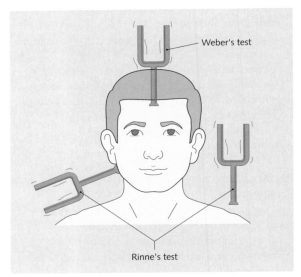

Fig. 18.6 Tuning fork tests. The tuning fork is placed on the vertex of the head in Weber's test. In Rinne's test a tuning fork is struck and placed close to the external ear or rested on the mastoid process.

- Deafness is commonly conductive (e.g., due to otitis media, ear wax).
- Sensory deafness can be further defined by formal audiometry to ascertain the frequency of loss.

Vertigo is most commonly peripheral. Central lesions (e.g., cerebellar lesions) are not associated

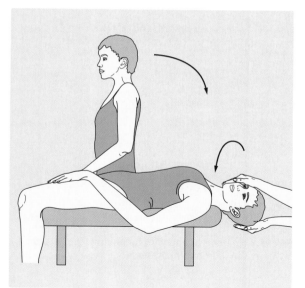

Fig. 18.7 Hallpike's manuever for testing positional nystagmus.

with deafness or tinnitus but are often associated with pronounced ataxia between the episodes of vertigo and persistent nystagmus.

Glossopharyngeal nerve (cranial nerve IX)
Function
The glossopharyngeal nerve has three functions:
- Sensory: taste for the posterior two-thirds of tongue, most of oropharynx, and soft palate.
- Parasympathetic.
- Motor: to stylopharyngeus.

Anatomy
The motor and sensory nuclei lie in the medulla. The nerve leaves the skull with the Xth and XIth nerves at the jugular foramen.

Examination
Gag reflex   Ask the patient to say "aah" with his or her mouth open and observe palatal movement. Touch the posterior wall of the oropharynx with a stick. This elicits constriction and elevation. If there is no response, ask the patient whether he or she felt the stimulus. The presence or absence of the gag reflex does not correlate with whether a patient has a safe swallow reflex after a CVA.

The gag reflex is unpleasant and should be performed only if a lesion of the IXth or Xth nerves is suspected.

Interpretation
The afferent limb is via the IXth nerve, the efferent from the Xth.

Vagus nerve (cranial nerve X)
Function
The vagus nerve supplies innervation to the viscera in the thorax and foregut as well as having smaller motor and sensory functions. The main functions are:
- Parasympathetic: visceral innervation to heart, lungs, foregut.
- Motor: to larynx, soft palate, pharynx.
- Sensory: for dura mater of the posterior cranial fossa, small part of the external ear.

Anatomy
The nucleus lies in the medulla.

Examination
Speech   Listen for dysphonia or a bovine cough associated with recurrent laryngeal nerve palsy.

Fig. 18.8 Assessment of tuning fork tests.

Assessment of tuning fork tests			
Condition	Rinne's (left ear)	Rinne's (right ear)	Weber's
normal hearing	positive	positive	heard in midline
conductive deficit in right ear	positive	negative	heard on right side
sensory deficit in right ear	positive	positive	heard on left side

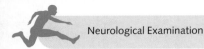
Soft palate Observe the uvula. In a unilateral lesion, it will droop away from the lesion.

Gag reflex See above for glossopharyngeal nerve.

Interpretation
In the presence of dysphonia, the vocal cords should be examined.

Accessory (spinal accessory) nerve (cranial nerve XI)
Function
The spinal accessory nerve is a motor nerve supplying the sternomastoid and trapezius muscles.

Anatomy
The anterior horn cells of the cervical cord innervate these muscles, but fibers pass up to the medulla before descending again through the jugular foramen.

Examination
Test the bulk and power of sternomastoid. Ask patients to:
- Force their chin downward against the resistance of your hand (bilateral).
- Turn chin to one side against resistance (unilateral weakness affects turning to the opposite side).

The power of trapezius can be tested by asking patients to shrug their shoulders against resistance.

Hypoglossal nerve (cranial nerve XII)
Function
The hypoglossal nerve is a motor nerve supplying innervation to the muscles of the tongue.

Anatomy
The nucleus is in the medulla.

Examination
Inspection Look at the tongue for wasting and fasciculation.

Protrusion Ask patients to protrude the tongue. If there is a unilateral lesion, the tongue will deviate toward the side of the lesion.

Motor function

When examining the motor system, the aim is to:
- Identify any lesions.
- Ascertain whether the lesion is an UMN or LMN lesion.

Features of UMN and LMN lesions	
UMN	**LMN**
no muscle wasting (but there may be disuse atrophy)	wasting
increased tone ("clasp-knife")	flaccid
weakness of characteristic distribution	marked weakness
hyperreflexia	depressed or absent reflex
abnormal plantar response	normal plantar response
no fasciculation	fasciculation

Fig. 18.9 Features of upper motor neuron (UMN) and lower motor neuron (LMN) lesions.

- Locate the anatomical site of the lesion.
- Consider the differential diagnosis of lesions at that site.

The fundamental distinction is between UMN (above the anterior horn cells) and LMN lesions (Fig. 18.9).

The examination should follow a strict routine of:
- Inspection.
- Palpation.
- Assessment of muscular tone.
- Assessment of power.
- Assessment of tendon reflexes (as part of the DTR exam).
- Assessment of coordination (as part of the cerebellar exam).
- Assessment of gait (as part of the cerebellar exam).

Inspection
Inspection should begin as the patient enters the examination room. Note posture, gait, coordination, abnormal movements, etc. The patient should be fully exposed on the examination table so that individual muscle groups can be observed. Inspect specifically for:
- Wasting: note symmetry; look specifically for distribution (e.g., proximal wasting).
- Fasciculation (spontaneous contraction of small groups of muscle fibers): usually implies a LMN lesion (e.g., motor neuron disease).

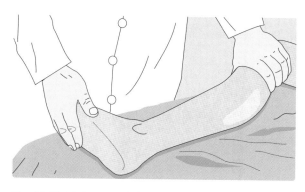

Fig. 18.10 Technique of eliciting ankle clonus. Bend the patient's knee slightly, supporting it with one hand. Grasp the forefoot with the other hand and suddenly dorsiflex the foot. Clonus is made up of regular oscillations of the foot. Sustained (>4 beats) clonus indicates an upper motor neuron (UMN) lesion. One or two beats is normal.

MRC classification of muscle power	
Grade	MRC grade of muscle strength
0	no movement
1	flicker of movement visible
2	movement possible with gravity eliminated
3	movement possible against gravity, but not resistance
4	movement possible against resistance, but weakened (often subdivided to 4−, 4, 4+)
5	normal power

Fig. 18.11 Medical Research Council (MRC) classification of muscle power.

- Tremors: note whether coarse and whether a resting tremor or an intention tremor.

Palpation

Palpate the muscle groups, specifically noting:
- Muscle bulk.
- Tenderness (e.g., myositis).

Assessment of muscular tone

Normally, there is a limited resistance through the range of movement.

 In assessing muscular tone it is essential that the patient is properly relaxed and lying in a neutral position.

If increased tone is suspected, attempt to elicit clonus (Fig. 18.10). Assessment of tone is subjective and requires experience, but specifically consider:
- Hypertonia: for example, "clasp-knife" (high resistance to initial movement and then sudden release; characteristic of UMN lesions), "lead-pipe rigidity" (resistance through the range of movement; in Parkinson's disease this in combination with the tremor produces "cogwheel rigidity").

- Hypotonia: for example, due to LMN and cerebellar lesions.

Assessment of power

Individual muscle groups should be tested to assess power. When testing, patients should be at a slight mechanical advantage so that if they have normal power, they can just overcome the resistance of the examiner. Muscle strength can be classified according to the Medical Research Council (MRC) grade (Fig. 18.11).

It is usually sufficient to test:
- Movements of the neck.
- Shoulder abduction and adduction.
- Movements of the elbows, wrists, and hands.
- Movements of the hips, knees, and ankle.

If you detect a weakness, it should be categorized as either UMN or LMN. If classified as LMN, the physical signs should be integrated to identify the lesion anatomically (Fig. 18.12).

When testing each muscle group, always consider:
- The myotome.
- The peripheral nerve supplying the muscles.

The major movements in the upper and lower limb are illustrated in Figs. 18.13 and 18.14. It is essential to be systematic if a weakness is identified, so that the pattern of involvement can be recognized as corresponding to a nerve root, peripheral nerve, or

Features of LMN lesions originating in the spinal cord, nerve root, peripheral nerve, neuromuscular junction, and muscle

Location of lesion	Examples	Features
anterior horn cells	motor neuron disease; polio	usually symmetrical; no myotome/nerve root distribution; often distal initially; no sensory involvement
nerve root (radiculopathy)	nerve root compression	distribution of affected muscles according to myotome; may have associated dermatomal sensory loss
peripheral nerve (neuropathy)	carpal tunnel	weakness according to nerve supply of affected nerve; usually associated sensory loss; early loss of reflexes
neuromuscular junction	myasthenia gravis	loss of power fluctuating in severity; not in distribution of peripheral nerve or myotome
muscle (myopathy)	n.a.	often has characteristic distribution of a particular disease; reflexes may be preserved early in disease; no sensory loss

Fig. 18.12 It is usually possible to localize a lower motor neuron (LMN) lesion as originating in the spinal cord, nerve root, peripheral nerve, neuromuscular junction, or muscle.

an individual muscle group (Fig. 18.15). This can be correlated with the other features of the examination of the peripheral nervous system.

Specific tests for the more common peripheral neuropathies are considered later.

Sensory function

Patients are usually aware of numbness, paresthesias, or altered sensation indicating a sensory pathology, but examination of the sensory system forms part of a routine assessment. Attempt to identify the modality of sensory loss and its distribution (e.g., correlating with a dermatome, peripheral nerve). A knowledge of the dermatomes is essential (Fig. 18.16).

Useful dermatomes to remember are: C5, deltoid; C6, thumb; C7, middle finger; C8, little finger; T4, nipple; T8, xiphoid; T10, umbilicus; T12, symphysis pubis; L4, medial leg; L5, between great and second toe; S1, lateral border of foot.

Light touch
Dab (do not stroke) the skin lightly with a small wisp of cotton wool. If there is decreased sensation, this should be mapped out. Start from the area of decreased sensation and move outward as this is more sensitive.

Pinprick
Use a disposable pin or needle gently and check that the patient can identify the stimulus as sharp. Temperature sensation is also conveyed in the spinothalamic tracts and is not routinely assessed.

Vibration
Place the base of a vibrating 128 Hz tuning fork on the distal phalanx of the great toe. Patients should be aware of a buzzing sensation. Ask patients to close their eyes and to indicate when they think that the tuning fork has stopped vibrating. Usually vibration sense is impaired peripherally. If absent, move proximally (i.e., from lateral malleolus to upper tibia and then iliac crest).

Loss of vibration sense is one of the earlier physical signs indicative of peripheral neuropathy in diabetes mellitus.

Fig. 18.13 The major muscle groups tested in an assessment of power in the upper limb. Patients should be at a slight mechanical advantage so that they can just overcome the resistance offered by the examiner.

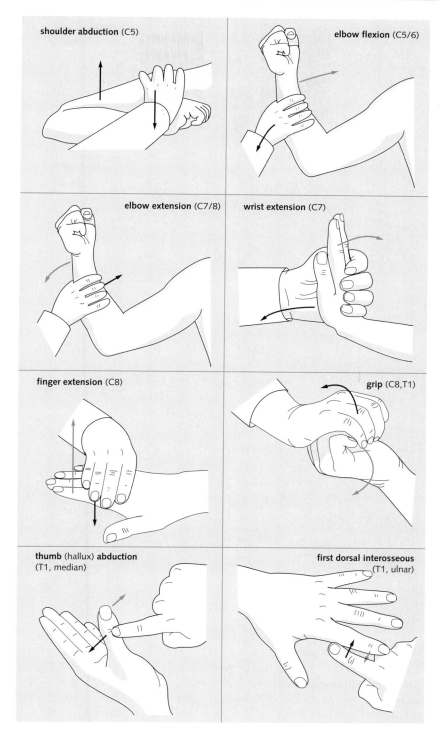

shoulder abduction (C5)

elbow flexion (C5/6)

elbow extension (C7/8)

wrist extension (C7)

finger extension (C8)

grip (C8,T1)

thumb (hallux) abduction (T1, median)

first dorsal interosseous (T1, ulnar)

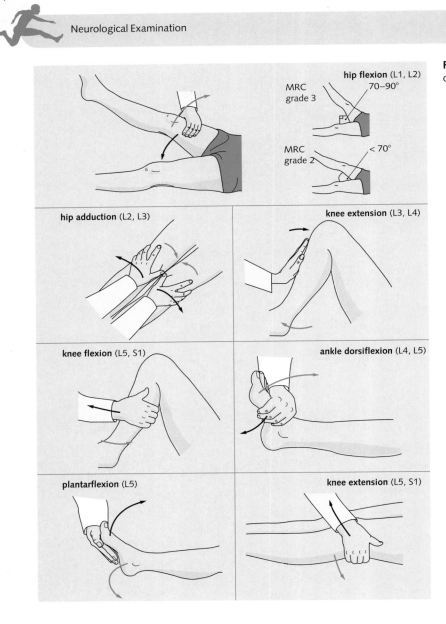

Fig. 18.14 Testing muscle groups of the lower limb.

Joint position sense

Start distally. Move the great toe passively, either extending or flexing, and observe whether the patient can identify the direction of movement. Be careful not to contact the second toe with your hand as this may give additional sensation to the patient. When you hold the toe, hold it by the side. This prevents the patient feeling the increase in pressure when moving the toe up or down. If there is impairment, test the ankle and knee.

Reflexes

The reflexes should be elicited using a reflex hammer. Compare the relative responses, both against normality and with each side. Make a note of the response—whether it appears normal, brisk, or reduced. If no response is obtained, try methods to reinforce the reflex. For example, ask patients to clench their teeth or hook their fingers around each other and try to separate their hands without disentangling their fingers (Fig. 18.17). The nerve

Nerve root, peripheral nerve, and muscle responsible for each movement			
Movement	Myotome	Peripheral nerve	Main muscle groups
shoulder abduction	C5, 6	axillary	deltoid
shoulder adduction	C5, 6, 7, 8	lateral pectoral, thoracodorsal	pectoralis major, latissimus dorsi
elbow flexion	C5, 6	musculocutaneous	biceps
elbow extension	C6, 7, 8	radial	triceps
wrist extension	C7, 8	radial	long extensors
wrist flexion	C8	ulnar and median	long flexors
pronation	C6, 7	median	pronator teres, pronator quadratus
supination	C6, 7	musculocutaneous, radial	biceps, supinator
finger abduction	T1	ulnar	dorsal interossei
finger adduction	T1	ulnar	
opposition of thumb	T1	median	opponens pollicis
extension of thumb at the interphalangeal joint	T1	radial	extensor pollicis longus
hip extension	L4, 5	inferior gluteal	glutei
hip flexion	L2, 3	femoral	iliopsoas
knee flexion	L5, S1	sciatic	hamstrings
knee extension	L2, 3, 4	femoral	quadriceps
dorsiflexion of foot	L4, 5	peroneal	tibialis anterior, long extensors, peroneus, extensor digitorum brevis
plantar flexion of foot	S1, 2	tibial	gastrocnemius, tibialis posterior
inversion of ankle	L4	peroneal, tibial	tibialis anterior, tibialis posterior
eversion of ankle	S1	peroneal	peronei, long extensors, extensor digitorum brevis
extension of great toe	L4, 5, S1	deep peroneal	extensor hallucis longus

Fig. 18.15 Nerve root, peripheral nerve, and muscle responsible for each movement. By integrating the pattern of weakness, it should be possible to recognize a pattern corresponding to these anatomical subdivisions.

roots of the more commonly elicited reflexes are listed in Fig. 18.18, and the reflex arc is shown in Fig. 18.19.

Disruption of the reflex may be due to a lesion at the level of the:
- Peripheral nerves (peripheral neuropathy). Typically the reflex is depressed early in the course of the pathology.
- Spinal cord.
- Neuromuscular junction.
- Muscle (myopathy). The reflex is usually retained until late in the natural history of the disease.

Cerebellar function

Assessment of coordination
Coordination in the upper limb is tested by the finger–nose test. Hold a finger at arm's length from patients and then ask them to rapidly touch the tip of their nose and then the tip of your finger with their index finger. The smoothness and accuracy of the movements should be interpreted and put into context with any muscle weakness.

The lower limbs may be assessed by the heel–chin test. Ask patients to place their right heel on their

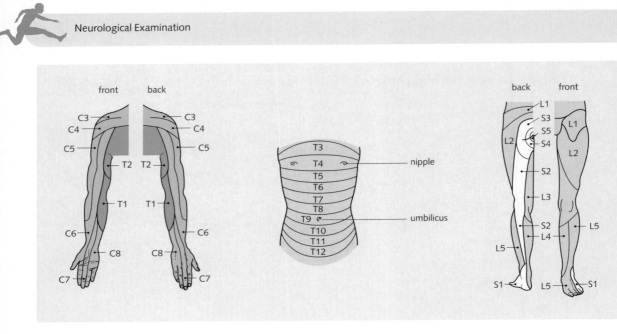

Fig. 18.16 Distribution of the dermatomes on the surface of the body.

left shin and to slide it down and up the shin, and then to repeat the test using the left heel.

If there is an intention tremor or dysmetria (irregular error in the distance and force of limb movements), cerebellar pathologies can be investigated by looking for dysdiadochokinesis. Ask patients to rapidly slap one palm with the other hand alternating between the palm and back of the hand.

Assessment of gait

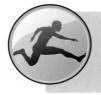 No neurological assessment is complete without an assessment of the patient's gait.

At a basic level, gait should be assessed as the patient walks into the examination room. Certain gaits are characteristic of certain pathologies. For example:

- Spastic gait: the extensor muscles are stiff and the foot is plantarflexed so that patients have a stiff gait and avoid catching their toes on the ground by circumducting the leg at the hips.

- Ataxia: the gait is wide-based and there is also marked clumsiness when patients are asked to walk in a straight line placing their heel immediately in front of the toe of the opposite foot (e.g., in cerebellar ataxia).
- High-stepping gait: in patients with foot drop, the foot is lifted high off the ground and then slapped back down.
- Parkinsonism: the gait is slow and shuffling with no associated arm swinging; patients often find it difficult to stop and turn around.
- Waddling gait: for example, due to proximal myopathy.

Romberg's test

Romberg's test may be positive if there is impaired position sense. Patients are asked to stand upright with their eyes closed. Marked swaying when patients close their eyes is "Rombergism" (Fig. 18.20).

Patterns of neurological damage

It is helpful when assessing neurological lesions to be aware of common patterns of deficits so that the anatomical site of the lesion can be determined (e.g., myopathy, peripheral neuropathy, nerve root, cortical

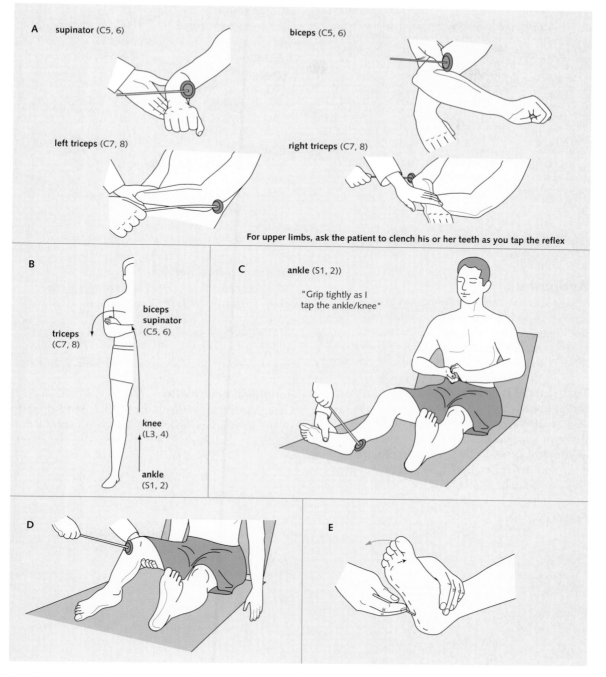

A supinator (C5, 6) biceps (C5, 6)

left triceps (C7, 8) right triceps (C7, 8)

For upper limbs, ask the patient to clench his or her teeth as you tap the reflex

B

triceps
(C7, 8)

biceps
supinator
(C5, 6)

knee
(L3, 4)

ankle
(S1, 2)

C ankle (S1, 2))

"Grip tightly as I
tap the ankle/knee"

D

E

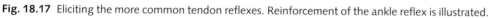

Fig. 18.17 Eliciting the more common tendon reflexes. Reinforcement of the ankle reflex is illustrated.

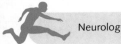

Nerve roots supplying the major reflexes	
Reflex	**Nerve root**
biceps	C5*, C6
brachioradialis	C6*, C7
triceps	C6, C7*, C8
knee	L2, L3*, L4*
ankle	S1, S2
anal	S2, S3, S4

Fig. 18.18 Nerve roots supplying the major reflexes. Asterisks indicate the major nerve root supplying each reflex.

lesion). Some of the more important lesions are described below.

Myopathy

Weakness and wasting of muscles occur in a distribution that is characteristic of the particular type of myopathy (e.g., facioscapulohumeral muscular dystrophy, Duchenne muscular dystrophy). Reflexes are preserved until the disease is advanced.

Peripheral nerves
Radial nerve

Damage to the radial nerve may cause wrist drop. Test sensation over the first dorsal interosseous muscle. Test extension of the interphalangeal joint of the thumb (e.g., compression neuropathy after sleeping with arm over a chair).

Median nerve

Damage to the median nerve (e.g., carpal tunnel syndrome) characteristically produces:
- Sensory loss over the palmar aspect of the lateral three and a half fingers.
- Wasting of the thenar eminence.
- Weakness of opposition, flexion, and abduction of the thumb.

Ulnar nerve

Ulnar nerve lesions (e.g., due to trauma at the elbow) result in:
- Sensory loss over the little finger and medial half of the ring finger.
- Wasting of the hypothenar eminence.
- Weakness of finger abduction and adduction.

Lateral popliteal nerve

The lateral popliteal nerve is sometimes damaged during a fracture to the head of the fibula. This may result in:
- Impaired sensation of the lateral calf.
- Foot drop.
- Weakness of dorsiflexion and eversion of the foot.

Peripheral neuropathy

Generalized neuropathy is usually in a "stocking and glove" distribution. Tendon reflexes are lost early in the course of disease.

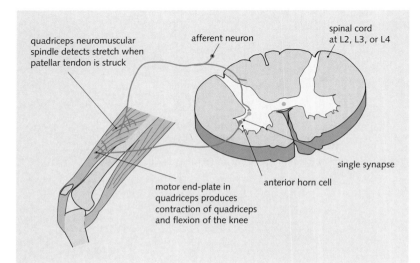

Fig. 18.19 Neurological pathway for the knee jerk.

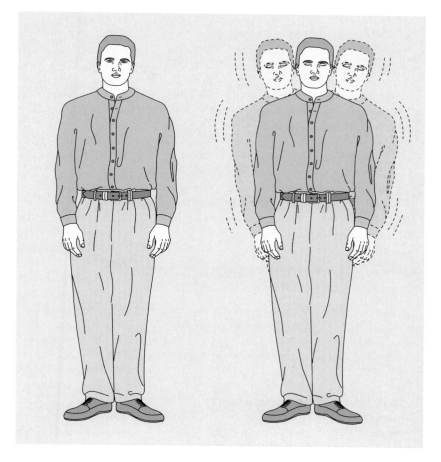

Fig. 18.20 Romberg's test. A positive test indicates impaired position sense. Patients can maintain a good posture when their eyes are open, but sway when asked to close their eyes.

Cerebellum

The main features of cerebellar pathology are:
- Gait ataxia (wide-based).
- Intention tremor.
- Dysdiadochokinesis.
- Nystagmus.
- Hypotonia.
- Dysmetria.
- Dysarthria ("staccato speech").

Extrapyramidal system

There is a wide range of extrapyramidal syndromes. They tend to be characterized by:
- Decreased movement (e.g., bradykinesia in Parkinson's disease).
- Involuntary movements (e.g., tardive dyskinesia with drug therapy).
- Rigidity.

Summary of neurological examination

In summary, when carrying out a neurological examination:
- It is of paramount importance to be systematic. Most of the signs represent a qualitative change from normality. This change can only be recognized with practice.
- Identifying a lesion is the easy part. A given lesion may be due to multiple pathologies at various locations in the nervous system. The next stage is to prepare a list of all the elicited signs and consider whether a single pathological lesion can account for them. If so, identify its anatomical site.
- Remember that lesions produce characteristic patterns of physical signs. For example, if a

weakness is identified, consider whether the pattern fits into a UMN or LMN pattern. If it is LMN, look for features that identify the site of the lesion (i.e., at the muscle itself, the neuromuscular junction, a peripheral nerve, a nerve root, or anterior horn cells). If the lesion is UMN in pattern, there are usually other localizing signs that allow identification of the anatomical point of pathology.

- Once the anatomical location of the lesion has been identified, prepare a differential diagnosis of possible pathologies that can produce a lesion at that site. Consider collateral information from the history or systemic examination to narrow down the differential diagnosis.

Stroke

Usually a diagnosis of stroke is apparent from the history, but the examination is crucial to confirm the presence of a focal neurological deficit, document baseline function objectively, and consider etiological factors.

Assess level of consciousness
See section on the unconscious patient (p. 170).

Define the neurological deficit
A full neurological assessment is essential to ascertain the degree of damage. It is often possible to identify the vascular territory affected. Occasionally, the lesion produces a more subtle lesion such as impaired cognition. The anatomical site of damage may offer prognostic information.

Consider etiology
The systemic examination may offer clues to the underlying cause.

Pulse
Arrhythmias, especially atrial fibrillation, predispose to emboli. Consider the possibility of a recent myocardial infarction, which may have caused a watershed infarct or been complicated by transient arrhythmias.

Blood pressure
Hypertension is one of the major risk factors for stroke. In the acute setting, it should be interpreted with caution and treated even more cautiously

because an abrupt drop in blood pressure may cause further ischemia since autoregulation will be impaired.

Eyes
Argyll Robertson pupils may suggest syphilis (now a rare cause of stroke in the U.S.) or diabetes mellitus.

Fundoscopy
Look for evidence of hypertensive and diabetic retinopathy.

Face
The facial appearance may suggest an underlying pathology, for example, plethora (polycythemia).

Neck
Listen carefully for a carotid bruit as a source of embolus. Have a low threshold for considering a Doppler scan of the carotid vessels as a patient with over 70% stenosis of the internal carotid artery may benefit from subsequent endarterectomy. Although detection of carotid bruits is not particularly sensitive, it is highly specific for the probability of significant stenosis.

Heart
Listen for any murmurs. Mitral stenosis (especially in association with atrial fibrillation) is a potent risk factor for left atrial thrombus and subsequent embolus. Consider the possibility of endocarditis (especially if there is a murmur). If there is fixed splitting of the second heart sound in association with a flow murmur, look for sources of paradoxical embolus from the venous circulation.

Epileptiform seizure

The diagnosis of epilepsy usually relies upon an objective eyewitness account. The doctor rarely sees a seizure in an individual patient.

Acute seizure
The priority is to insure that patients do not harm themselves and then to assess and if necessary provide specific therapy for the seizure. One should:
- Protect the airway.
- Insure that the patient will not harm him or herself.

Fig. 18.21 Assessment of a patient during a seizure may reveal the presence of a condition other than typical epilepsy.

Assessment of a patient during a seizure to reveal conditions other than typical epilepsy	
Cause of collapse	**Discriminatory features**
syncope	usually apparent from prodromal history; check pulse rate (e.g., tachyarrhythmia, Stokes–Adams attack); check postural blood pressure; pallor during episode
narcolepsy	no convulsions; patient rousable
hysteria	often many atypical features; usually only occur when there is an audience; no urinary incontinence/tongue biting

- Observe the nature of the seizure activity (e.g., tonic–clonic, focal, absence attack).
- Check pulse rate and, if possible, blood pressure.
- Check blood sugar, obtain blood for electrolytes (toxins).
- If seizure is prolonged, undertake measures for status epilepticus.

Postictal period

Usually the patient is seen in the postictal period, having been brought to the hospital after collapsing. The history is central to the diagnosis (see Epileptic seizure, p. 60), and very often the examination is unremarkable. The examination may be useful for considering the differential diagnosis or for assessing the etiology and functional consequences of the seizure (Fig. 18.21). Remember, any neurological symptoms may be observed after a seizure, but they should be monitored and seen to resolve.

Perform detailed neurological assessment

In particular, focus on:
- Level of consciousness. Check the Glasgow Coma Score (Fig. 18.22) until a normal level of consciousness is achieved as seizure may be the presentation of head injury or intracranial bleed.
- Paralysis. A postictal focal weakness (Todd's paralysis) may be present for 24 hours following a seizure, but consider the presence of an acute CVA or intracranial space-occupying lesion if neurological signs are present.
- Eyes. Check pupillary responses and fundoscopy to exclude papilledema.

Glasgow Coma Score	
Eyes (E)	
open spontaneously (with blinking)	4
open to command of speech	3
open in response to pain (applied to limbs or sternum)	2
not opening	1
Motor function (M)	
obeys commands	6
localizes to pain	5
withdraws from pain	4
flexor response to pain (decorticate)	3
extensor response to pain (decerebrate)	2
no response to pain	1
Vocalization (V)	
appropriate speech	5
confused speech	4
inappropriate words	3
groans only	2
no speech	1

Fig. 18.22 The Glasgow Coma Score.

Perform systemic examination to identify precipitating cause

It is particularly important to perform a detailed systemic examination to try to identify an underlying cause for the epileptic seizure so that specific therapy may be offered. Consider:
- Alcohol withdrawal (common): signs of chronic liver disease, smell of alcohol on breath, unkempt condition.
- Trauma.

169

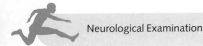

- Pyrexia (infants).
- Encephalitis: fever, level of consciousness, focal neurological signs, herpetic ulcer.
- Malignancy: look for signs of primary bronchial, breast, colonic, or kidney tumor.
- Degenerative brain disease (e.g., dementia).

Unconscious patient

Assess level of consciousness

The Glasgow Coma Score (GCS) is widely used to provide a simple reproducible objective assessment of conscious level. This is based on the best responses obtained (Fig. 18.22). If you don't have time to assess the GCS, use the AVPU scoring system: is the patient Alert, does the patient respond to Voice, does the patient respond to Pain, or is the patient Unresponsive?

The Glasgow Coma Score is particularly useful if repeated observations are made so that a rapid and unambiguous diagnosis of a deteriorating level of consciousness can be made.

Perform full neurological examination

Look for any localizing signs. Pay particular attention to:
- Pupil size and response to light (Fig. 18.23) (including symmetry). Some drugs (e.g., opiates) constrict pupils; other drugs (e.g., phenothiazines, amphetamines) dilate pupils. "Coning" results in a single fixed dilated pupil; pontine lesions result in pinpoint pupils; brain death results in fixed dilated pupils.
- Fundi (especially for papilledema).
- Gag and corneal reflexes.
- Motor responses.
- Tendon reflexes.
- Abnormal tone.

Perform detailed systemic examination

The six traumatic things that kill you quickly and can be treated are best remembered as ATOM FC:

A = Airways obstruction
T = Tension pneumothorax
O = Open pneumothorax
M = Massive hemothorax
F = Flailed chest
C = Cardiac tamponade.

Cosma may be due to metabolic or infective cause, cardiovascular pathology, or other causes. In particular note:
- Evidence of trauma or head injury (look for otorrhea or cerebrospinal fluid leaking from the nose).
- Temperature (e.g., hypothyroidism, infection).
- Evidence of needle marks (indicating diabetes mellitus or drug addiction).
- Jaundice or other features of chronic liver disease.
- Breath (e.g., revealing alcohol, diabetic ketoacidosis).
- Respiratory pattern (e.g., Cheyne–Stokes respiration, Kussmaul's respirations of diabetes mellitus or uremia).
- Cyanosis (e.g., due to hypoxia).

Exclude hypoglycemia or hyperglycemia early in the assessment of an unconscious patient by performing a finger blood glucose analysis.

Multiple sclerosis

Multiple sclerosis causes neurological lesions that are disseminated in time and place. It can be diagnosed with reasonable confidence from the history of relapses and remissions and thorough examination if it follows a typical course. Areas of demyelination may occur anywhere in the central nervous system, but certain patterns are more common.

Sites of involvement

The more common sites of involvement are:
- Optic nerve (optic neuritis).
- Brainstem.
- Cerebellum.
- Cervical cord.
- Periventricular region.

Fig. 18.23 Examination of the pupils in an unconscious patient. Note the size and reaction to light. In addition, note the position of gaze fixation. (*Looking towards the lesion; **looking away from the lesion; †normally if the head is held and turned quickly from side to side the eyes swivel in the opposite direction to the head.)

small/pinpoint pupils	opiates, pontine lesion (hemorrhage/ischemia/compression)
large fixed pupils	tricyclic antidepressant or sedative overdose, eyedrops, atropine, and death
unilateral dilated fixed pupils	supratentorial mass lesion
mid-position fixed pupils	midbrain lesion
congugate gaze to one side	cerebral lesion on that side* or contralateral pontine lesion**
dysconjugate eye movement	drug overdose, brainstem lesion
abnormal doll's eye movement — direction of turn — normal / abnormal	the eyes move "with the head" with a brainstem lesion†

Differential diagnosis of optic atrophy	
Site of lesion	**Causes**
retina	central retinal occlusion; toxic (e.g., quinine, methylated spirits)
optic nerve	optic and retrobulbar neuritis (e.g., multiple scierosis); chronic glaucoma; any cause of papilledema; toxin (e.g., alcohol, tobacco, ethambutol); tumor (e.g., meningioma, optic glioma)
optic chiasm	pituitary tumor; craniopharyngioma; meningioma

Fig. 18.24 Differential diagnosis of optic atrophy.

Eyes

Certain patterns of disease should be distinguished:

- Retrobulbar neuritis: relative afferent pupillary defect, central scotoma.
- Optic neuritis: also note swelling of the optic disk acutely and temporal pallor following recovery.
- Optic atrophy: a common finding in longstanding multiple sclerosis but should be distinguished from other pathologies (Fig. 18.24).

- Nystagmus: often jerking or ataxic; pronounced in late disease.
- Internuclear ophthalmoplegia: diplopia on lateral gaze due to failure of adducting eye to cross midline and demyelination of medial longitudinal bundle.

Brainstem

Multiple brainstem or cerebellar signs may be present, especially nystagmus, diplopia, intention tremor, scanning speech.

Spinal cord

Spastic paraparesis is common in late disease. Other signs can include bladder dysfunction, decreased limb sensation, and loss of posture sensibility, which is often marked.

Mental signs

Both euphoria and depression or irritability are common.

Always attempt to make a functional assessment of how multiple sclerosis might affect daily activities.

19. Endocrine Examination

Inspection
Note weight and height. Calculate the patient's body mass index (BMI); diabetic control may improve with a normal BMI.

Macrovascular complications
Ischemic heart disease and cerebrovascular disease
Diabetics have a much increased risk of stroke and ischemic heart disease. It is important to modify any reversible risk factors. Assess these other risk factors, especially:

- Obesity: obesity is not only a risk factor for macrovascular disease but also predisposes to poor glycemic control.
- Blood pressure control.
- Smoking; nicotine staining of fingers and hair.
- Xanthoma, arcus senilis: hyperlipidemia.

Peripheral vascular disease
Examine the peripheral pulses (femoral, popliteal, dorsalis pedis, and posterior tibial arteries). Consider measuring the ratio of ankle/brachial artery pressure. Listen for bruits, especially over the abdomen and carotid and femoral arteries, which indicate turbulent flow and are suggestive of stenosis.

Look for evidence of ulcers, including between the toes. Ulcers may be painless and large without patients knowing that they have one.

Microvascular complications
Eyes
Examination of the eyes is important in diabetic patients because they are at risk for many diseases. Diabetic patients should have a detailed fundoscopic assessment with dilated pupils at least once a year.

Note the following:
- Cataracts: more common in diabetics.
- Evidence of background retinopathy ("dot and blot" hemorrhages, exudates).
- Proliferative retinopathy (neovascularization, vitreous hemorrhage).
- Macular edema.

Assess eye movements (especially in longstanding diabetes mellitus) for a third nerve palsy due to mononeuritis multiplex.

Check visual acuity, which is often reduced due to maculopathy.

Peripheral neuropathy
Test for evidence of a "stocking and glove" sensory loss. Loss of vibration and joint position sense are often the first modalities to be affected, especially in the legs. A defined peripheral nerve (e.g., median nerve) lesion (mononeuritis multiplex) may also be present.

Diabetic nephropathy
Nephropathy is particularly common in the presence of retinopathy and neuropathy. It is also a marker for an increased risk of ischemic heart disease. Look for proteinuria. If urinalysis is negative for protein, test the urine for microalbumin. This should be done yearly.

Urinalysis is an essential component of examination of the diabetic patient!

Feet
The feet of diabetic patients should be examined at every examination. Look at general foot care such as the presence of ulcers and the state of the nails. Test the temperature, pulses, and shape of the foot to determine vascular and neuropathic causes. The presence of abnormally sited callosities on the sole may indicate uneven weight distribution.

Assess diabetic control
Different patients use different methods for recording glucose control.

Urinalysis
Based on the renal threshold for glucose and the availability of fingerstick testing for blood glucose, the urinalysis has little role in testing for glucose.

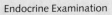

Fingerstick blood glucose testing

Look at the patient's own record of blood glucose assessments. Many of the meters have a recall function that allows you to retrieve the patient's blood glucose values. This is most informative in type 1 diabetes mellitus. You may wish to ask patients to perform an estimate in front of you so that you can assess their technique.

Evidence of skin infections (e.g., boils, abscesses, candidiasis) may suggest chronically poor control.

Assess injection sites

Look for complications such as scarring, abscesses, and lipodystrophy, which result from not rotating injection sites frequently enough. Note any amyotrophy (painful wasting of a muscle group, e.g., quadriceps).

Diabetic coma

A young patient may present with diabetes and diabetic ketoacidosis. Any treated patient may have hypoglycemia complicating therapy.

 If there is any doubt about the cause of a coma in a diabetic patient and the glucose level is not known, treat with intravenous glucose first.

Diabetic ketoacidosis (DKA)

DKA typically occurs in a younger person. In particular:

- Note the respiratory pattern. Kussmaul's respiration suggests acidosis ("air hunger").
- Note the mental state. The patient may be alert but usually confused or stuporous.
- Smell the breath. Ketones may be detectable.
- Consider fluid status. The patient with dry skin and mucous membranes, decreased (or undetectable) jugular venous pressure (JVP), and hypotension is invariably dehydrated.
- Consider the underlying cause.
- Fever is often absent before therapy, even in the presence of infection, but sources of infection should be carefully sought.
- Do arterial blood gases. Patients can be extremely acidotic, and this needs to be monitored.

Most centers now have DKA protocols. Know where to find yours and have a look at it before you start working there.

Hyperosmolar nonketotic coma

Hyperosmolar nonketotic coma usually presents in a similar fashion as DKA, but in elderly and middle-aged subjects. Many of the clinical signs are the same, as are the basic management strategies:

- Rehydrate.
- Optimize acid–base balance.
- Replace insulin deficiency.
- Look for and treat the underlying cause.
- Provide general supportive care.

The management differs only in the fine tuning.

Hyperthyroidism

Like hypothyroidism (see below), many systems may show signs of hyperthyroidism, and although marked hyperthyroidism due to Graves' disease is unmistakable, the signs are often nonspecific. Hyperthyroidism occurs in the differential diagnosis of many symptoms and signs.

Inspection

General inspection often provides clues that are easily overlooked (Fig. 19.1). In particular, note:

- General demeanor: patients are typically agitated, restless, and irritable with poor concentration.
- Facies (e.g., exophthalmos).
- Goiter: associated with Graves' disease, toxic multinodular goiter.

Cardiovascular system

Cardiovascular abnormalities are common in thyroid disease and may provide a sensitive measure of assessing thyroid status in a treated patient. Look for the presence of:

- Tachycardia (very common).
- Atrial fibrillation: although this is a common arrhythmia, its presence should always raise a suspicion of hyperthyroidism. This is important because hyperthyroidism is an easily treatable cause of atrial fibrillation.
- Warm, vasodilated peripheries with a bounding arterial pulse.
- Hypertension: occasionally a feature.
- Ischemic heart disease.
- Mitral valve disease (especially mitral stenosis).

Fig. 19.1 Symptoms and signs of hyperthyroidism.

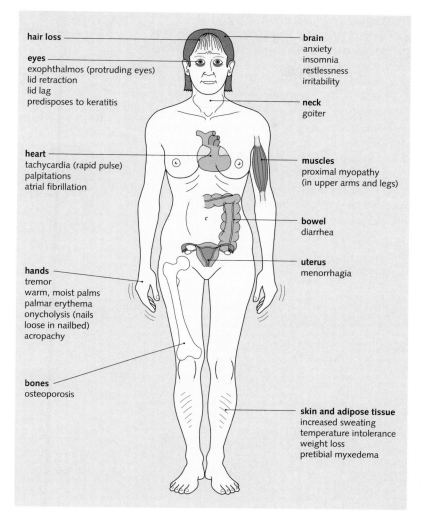

hair loss

eyes
exophthalmos (protruding eyes)
lid retraction
lid lag
predisposes to keratitis

heart
tachycardia (rapid pulse)
palpitations
atrial fibrillation

hands
tremor
warm, moist palms
palmar erythema
onycholysis (nails
loose in nailbed)
acropachy

bones
osteoporosis

brain
anxiety
insomnia
restlessness
irritability

neck
goiter

muscles
proximal myopathy
(in upper arms and legs)

bowel
diarrhea

uterus
menorrhagia

skin and adipose tissue
increased sweating
temperature intolerance
weight loss
pretibial myxedema

 The presence of atrial fibrillation in any patient should provoke a search for the underlying cause.

Neurological system

A brief examination often reveals discriminatory signs. For example:

- Fine resting tremor.
- Agitated, restless, hyperactive, shaky, irritable mental state. The patient may have a frank psychosis.
- Proximal myopathy, which may be profound.

Features to suggest Graves' disease
Eye signs

Graves' disease is particularly associated with eye signs, which can be used to differentiate it from other causes of hyperthyroidism. Note the presence of:

- Lid lag: upper eyelid does not keep pace with the eyeball as it traces a finger moving downward from above.
- Exophthalmos.
- Chemosis.
- Ophthalmoplegia: extraocular muscles become swollen and develop secondary fibrotic changes.
- Proptosis: hyperthyroidism is the most common cause of unilateral and bilateral proptosis.

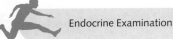

Pretibial myxedema, thyroid acropachy, and features to suggest general autoimmune predisposition

Deposition of mucopolysaccharides in the subcutaneous tissues of the legs produces a nontender infiltration on the front of the shins. Occasionally, it can present acutely.

Thyroid acropachy is a syndrome resembling clubbing with new bone formation in the fingers. It is classically associated with exophthalmos and pretibial myxedema.

Thyroid disease is associated with other autoimmune processes. In particular, look for alopecia and vitiligo.

Hypothyroidism

Hypothyroidism often develops insidiously and nonspecifically, especially in the elderly. A keen level of awareness is important, and the diagnosis is often made by an observant doctor who has never seen the patient previously.

 It is very easy to overlook a diagnosis of hypothyroidism. Always maintain a high index of suspicion, especially if the patient is seen on a regular basis.

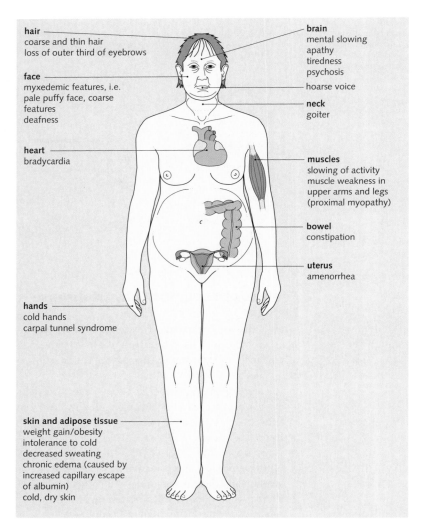

hair
coarse and thin hair
loss of outer third of eyebrows

face
myxedemic features, i.e. pale puffy face, coarse features
deafness

heart
bradycardia

hands
cold hands
carpal tunnel syndrome

skin and adipose tissue
weight gain/obesity
intolerance to cold
decreased sweating
chronic edema (caused by increased capillary escape of albumin)
cold, dry skin

brain
mental slowing
apathy
tiredness
psychosis
hoarse voice

neck
goiter

muscles
slowing of activity
muscle weakness in upper arms and legs (proximal myopathy)

bowel
constipation

uterus
amenorrhea

Fig. 19.2 Symptoms and signs of hypothyroidism.

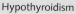

Inspection

It is easy to overlook hypothyroidism, so always consider the diagnosis, especially for patients presenting with chronic fatigue, dementia, slow thought, or nonspecific difficulty coping with previously simple tasks (Fig. 19.2).

Note the:

- Facies.
- Body shape: obesity, which is usually mild.
- Presence of a goiter: for example, if due to Hashimoto's thyroiditis, iodine deficiency.
- Nonpitting edema.
- Dry scaly skin.

Cardiovascular system

Discriminatory features may include:

- Cold peripheries.
- Bradycardia: a useful sign, especially if it is out of context with the patient's condition.
- Hypothermia.
- Pericardial effusion (i.e., difficult to locate apex beat, quiet heart sounds), heart failure.

Neurological system

It is common to find neurological signs, for example:

- Slow-relaxing deep tendon reflexes (classically at the ankle joint).
- Proximal myopathy.
- Carpal tunnel syndrome.
- Deep, hoarse voice.
- Mental slowing, which may present with dementia, stupor, or even coma.

Slow-relaxing reflexes are a particularly useful sign for confirming a clinical suspicion of hypothyroidism.

20. Reticuloendothelial Examination

Overview

Examination of lymph node groups is important in many disease states. It is important to know the anatomical drainage pattern of the major organs because regional lymphadenopathy may be the first manifestation of local disease.

Normally, lymph nodes are not palpable, except in some thin people. If a single lymph node is found to be enlarged, it is important to adopt a systematic approach.

Examination routine

How to examine any lump

You need to expose the area in question and then:

Inspect

Look at the shape of the lump and its position. Is there any associated color change or change in the skin overlying the lump? Remember to ask if the lump is painful before:

Palpation

Ask yourself whether there is any difference in temperature between the lump and the surrounding area. Feel and measure the shape, size (length, width, and depth), and surface.

- Determine the edge of the lump. Is it well or poorly demarcated? What is the consistency of the lump?
- Is it pulsatile? If so, is it expansile, or is it a transmitted pulse?
- Is the lump compressible or even reducible? (e.g., a form of hernia). Is a cough impulse present?
- Is a fluid thrill present in the lump, or is it fluctuant?
- Now try moving the lump. What is it fixed to? Is it in the skin, or is it fixed to muscle?

Auscultate

You should listen over the lump for both bowel sounds and bruits. Lastly, try to transilluminate the lump to see if it is fluid-filled. You may need to switch off the light to get a clear idea.

Now that you've finished with the lump, examine the surrounding tissue. Is there any change in strength or sensation?

Examine all lymph node groups

Examine all lymph node groups systematically to define the anatomical distribution of the enlarged lymph nodes (Fig. 20.1). It is also important to examine the liver and spleen, both of which are reticuloendothelial organs and may be enlarged in the presence of generalized lymphadenopathy.

Define the characteristics of the enlarged lymph node(s)

Define the texture, size, mobility, and fixation to superficial and other tissues of the enlarged lymph node(s) (as with the examination of any lump). Certain characteristics are suggestive of different disease processes. For example:

- Rubbery texture is suggestive of lymphoma.
- Hard, matted, fixed lymph nodes suggest malignancy.
- Tender lymph nodes suggest infection or other inflammatory state.

Explore the region drained by the enlarged lymph node group

If a single lymph node group is enlarged, try to identify the cause. The broad causes of lymphadenopathy are:

- Infection.
- Metastatic tumor.
- Lymphoproliferative disorder.
- Sarcoidosis.

In cases of cellulitis or other bacterial infection, it is sometimes possible to see lymphangitis. It is visible as thin, red streaks following the line of the lymphatics in the skin.

Perform a systemic examination

Consider the pathological cause by performing a systemic examination, concentrating on inflammatory or malignant conditions draining into that lymph node group. Consider the more common causes of localized and systemic lymphadenopathy (Fig. 20.2).

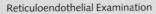

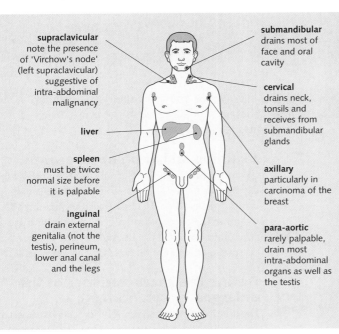

supraclavicular
note the presence of 'Virchow's node' (left supraclavicular) suggestive of intra-abdominal malignancy

liver

spleen
must be twice normal size before it is palpable

inguinal
drain external genitalia (not the testis), perineum, lower anal canal and the legs

submandibular
drains most of face and oral cavity

cervical
drains neck, tonsils and receives from submandibular glands

axillary
particularly in carcinoma of the breast

para-aortic
rarely palpable, drain most intra-abdominal organs as well as the testis

Fig. 20.1 Position of the major lymph node groups and lymphoid organs.

Differential diagnosis of localized and generalized lymphadenopathy		
	Lymphadenopathy	**Features and examples**
localized	infection (bacterial, viral, fungal)	pharyngitis, dental (cervical); lymphogranuloma venereum (inguinal)
	lymphoma (Hodgkin's, non-Hodgkin's)	can present anywhere, but cervical group is the most common
	malignancy	Virchow's node (left supraclavicular lymphadenopathy due to intra-abdominal or thoracic disease); breast cancer (axillary or supraclavicular)
generalized	infection	infectious mononucleosis; syphilis; tuberculosis; toxoplasmosis; HIV
	malignancy	lymphoma; leukemia (especially CLL); carcinoma (unusual)
	autoimmune disease	SLE, rheumatoid arthritis, sarcoidosis, other connective tissue diseases
	drugs	
	hyperthyroidism	

Fig. 20.2 Differential diagnosis of localized and generalized lymphadenopathy. SLE, systemic lupus erythematosus.

Usually the cause of lymphadenopathy is apparent from a detailed history and systemic examination, but if further investigation is needed, the most useful tests include:
• Full blood count and review of smear: for infection, leukemia.

• Erythrocyte sedimentation rate (ESR) and C-reactive protein (CRP): for malignancy, systemic inflammatory disease, systemic lupus erythematosus (SLE). These are markers of an acute inflammatory response, and a differential rise in ESR or CRP is occasionally discriminatory.

Fig. 20.3 Some dermatological terms.

Some dermatological terms	
alopecia	absence of hair where it normally grows
bulla	a circumscribed elevation of skin greater than 5 mm containing fluid
crusting	scale composed of either dried fluid or blood
erythema	a flushing of the skin due to the dilatation of the capillaries
excoriation	an erosion or ulcer secondary to scratching
lichenification	thickening of the epidermis of the skin with exaggeration of the normal creases
macule	small flat area of altered skin color or texture
nodule	a solid mass in the skin greater than 5 mm
papule	a small solid elevation of skin less than 5 mm
petechia	pinhead-sized flat collection of blood in the skin
plaque	elevation area of skin greater than 20 mm without depth
purpura	a large flat or raised collection of blood in the skin
pustule	visible accumulation of pus in the skin
ulcer	a loss in the continuity of an epithelially lined surface
vesicle	circumscribed elevation of skin less than 5 mm, containing fluid

- Biochemical profile, especially liver function.
- Chest radiography: for example, for sarcoid, malignancy, chest infection.
- Viral screens, autoantibody profiles, blood culture.
- Lymph node biopsy: often provides diagnostic information if sinister pathology is suspected.

If a single lymph node is enlarged, explore the region drained by that lymph node in detail. Regional lymphadenopathy is common, but usually transient. Persistent lymphadenopathy always warrants investigation.

Skin examination

The skin is the single largest organ in the body and yet is often overlooked. Rashes are common things to be asked about, and you need to be able to describe the lesion even if you cannot make a precise diagnosis so that you can communicate with others about it. Differing institutions have differing expectations about which terms they expect students to be familiar with (Fig. 20.3). During your dermatology rotation they should provide you with a dictionary of what they expect. Try to assimilate some of it!

When examining a rash, you will need to expose the patient in a well-lit room. The patient may well be shy about the lesion and feel that it is unsightly, so be sensitive. Have a chaperone present. First consider the distribution of the rash. Take a step back and look. Is it only on areas exposed to sunlight? Is it dermatomal in distribution (e.g., herpes zoster)? Is it related to jewellery or buttons? Is the rash generalized or localized, bilateral or unilateral? Are any areas spared?

Next, what is the morphology of the lesion? You need your dictionary to help with terminology. Try and determine the shape, size, color, and margins of any lesions you can see. If you cannot remember the special phrase, just describe exactly what you see in plain English.

21. Breast Examination

Examination routine

Breast examination forms an integral part of a full examination. However, a more detailed breast examination is always necessary if the presenting symptoms:

- Are breast symptoms (e.g., lump, pain, nipple discharge, change in appearance).
- Arouse suspicion of disseminated malignancy with an undiagnosed primary (e.g., presentation with pleural effusion, hepatomegaly, bony tenderness).
- Include fever of unknown cause.

As with any system, a methodical approach is needed. Anticipate what information might be obtained from each part of the examination and how each elicited sign is placed into context with the presenting illness.

Patient exposure and position

Great sensitivity is essential. Very often the patient feels uncomfortable or embarrassed, especially if the doctor is male. Remember that many patients are terrified, not only of the examination, but of the potential underlying diagnosis. It is not uncommon for women to "ignore" a breast mass for several months or even years.

Explain clearly why the examination is being performed and the useful information that is likely to be gained. Insure complete privacy. It is clearly unacceptable for another doctor, student, or nurse to burst through the door, revealing a semiclad patient to the waiting room or ward! The room should be warm, and a blanket should always be provided so that the patient can remain covered until the examination is performed.

Explain clearly what the examination will entail before asking the patient to undress. Ask the patient to remove all clothing (including bra) from the waist upwards, and to sit on the side of the examination table. You must have a female chaperone with you at all times.

The examination follows the usual sequence of:
- Inspection.
- Palpation.
- Systemic examination.

Inspection

Remember to look at the whole patient. Make a mental note of:

- Age. Breast carcinoma is more common in older women but can occur in any age group from the third decade onward. Fibroadenoma is more common in premenopausal women. Abscess is much more common in women of childbearing age.
- Sex. Men also get breast disease!
- General health.

Breast substance

Ask patients to sit still facing you with arms by their side (Fig. 21.1) and with arms raised above their head. A mass tethered to the skin may then become apparent, and the undersurface of the breasts can be seen. Note:

- Symmetry. It is not uncommon for one breast to be slightly larger than the other, but underlying masses, infections, or nipple disease can also cause asymmetry of size, shape, or nipples.
- Any obvious mass.
- Skin discoloration. Infections and occasionally malignancy may cause a red discoloration.
- Skin puckering or "peau d'orange" (Fig. 21.2). Peau d'orange is caused by infiltration of the skin lymphatic system, and as the name implies, its appearance resembles the peel of an orange.

Nipples

Inspect the nipples carefully, especially noting the following:

- Symmetry.
- Retraction or deviation. If one or both nipples are retracted, ask the patient if this is a new phenomenon. This is an ominous sign. As well as carcinoma, it is associated with chronic abscess and fat necrosis.
- Discharge. If present, note whether it appears milky (galactorrhea), bloody, or pustular.

183

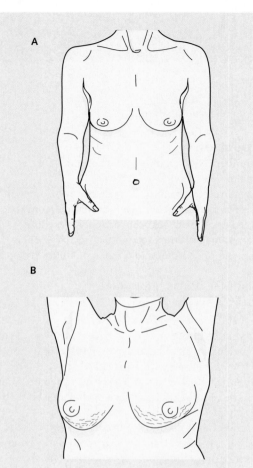

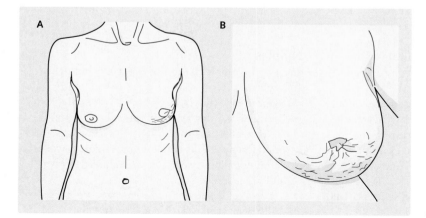

• Skin color. Particularly note the presence of an eczematous rash suggestive of Paget's disease of the nipple.

Palpation

The normal consistency of a breast varies considerably. It is recommended to start the examination with palpation of the normal breast. Palpate with the palmar surface of the fingers. It is helpful to divide the breast into quadrants (Fig. 21.3). Palpate each quadrant in turn, noting:

• Consistency and texture of the breast.
• Tenderness.
• Presence of any mass.

Palpation can also be performed radially (like the spokes of a wheel) or in increasing concentric circles.

Examine the breast with symptoms. Before palpating, ask patients to point to the area of tenderness or to any lump that they may have felt. Once again, examine each quadrant in turn. If a mass is felt, it should be systematically examined as described below.

Breast mass

If any lump or mass is identified on systemic examination, the essential features should be described. This is well illustrated with a breast mass. The following characteristics should be noted.

Fig. 21.1 (A) Ask the patient to sit facing you with hands on hips. (B) Then ask the patient to lift her arms in the air. Skin tethering may become apparent, and abnormalities on the undersurface of the breast will become visible.

Fig. 21.2 Inspection often reveals obvious asymmetry. (A) A retracted nipple and skin tethering on the left breast. (B) Peau d'orange in association with a retracted nipple.

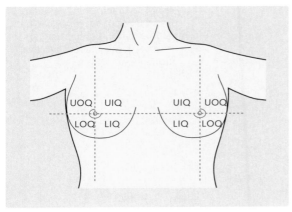

Fig. 21.3 Quadrants of the breast. Upper outer quadrant (UOQ), upper inner quadrant (UIQ), lower outer quadrant (LOQ), lower inner quadrant (LIQ).

Position

It is usual to describe a breast mass in relation to the quadrant in which it is located. A breast carcinoma is more common in the upper outer quadrant. Remember to palpate the axillary tail, which also contains breast tissue.

Size

Describe the size of the mass in three dimensions. Ideally measure the mass objectively with a tape measure or calipers to decrease interobserver error. This is essential to assessing the progression or regression of a lesion (e.g., judging the response of breast carcinoma to chemotherapy).

Consistency

Note the consistency of any mass. In practice, it is easiest to use terms such as:
- Craggy: literally like a rock.
- Hard: like pressing on your forehead.
- Rubbery: like pressing on the tip of your nose.
- Soft: like pressing on your lips.

Relation to the skin

Note the presence of tethering or fixation to the skin. Fixation suggests an infiltrating carcinoma; tethering occurs in carcinoma, abscess, or fat necrosis.

Relation to underlying tissue

Note the mobility of any lump. A mass fixed to deeper tissue is much more likely to be a carcinoma.

Fibroadenomas are typically described as highly mobile and may be difficult to palpate. Trapping a

fibroadenoma between finger and thumb can be tricky, and has been likened to chasing a mouse.

Tenderness

Breast carcinoma is rarely tender on presentation. A tender mass is much more likely to be an abscess, cyst, or fat necrosis.

Skin discoloration

Note any change in the appearance of the skin overlying the mass. Erythema is common in association with infections. Paget's disease of the nipple presents with an eczematous rash, a carcinoma occasionally has a red or blue hue.

Temperature

Inflammatory lesions often produce palpable warmth.

Associated lesions

It is essential to examine the rest of the breast for the presence of a second mass. It is not rare for breast carcinoma to present with bilateral disease. Fibroadenosis often presents with multiple lumps.

If breast carcinoma is suspected, a full systemic examination is essential. Look for evidence of metastatic spread. In particular, check for the presence of:
- Hepatomegaly: liver metastases result in a grim prognosis; note the presence of jaundice.
- Pleural effusion: the lung is a common site of metastatic spread.
- Bony tenderness: bony metastases are the most common site of secondary breast malignancy after axillary lymph nodes, and the axial skeleton is often involved. Disease may be present for several years.
- Ascites: peritoneal deposits often present with ascites.

Lymphatic drainage

Palpation of the axillary lymph nodes forms part of the routine breast examination (see below).

An example of a recording of the presence of a breast mass in the medical notes is illustrated in Fig. 21.4.

Axillary examination

Breast examination is incomplete without examination of the axilla because they are the natural site of lymphatic drainage of breast tissue. Inspect the axilla for any obvious lumps.

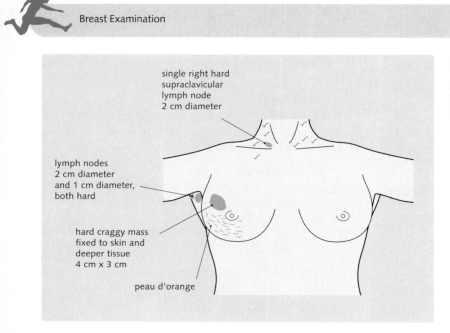

single right hard
supraclavicular
lymph node
2 cm diameter

lymph nodes
2 cm diameter
and 1 cm diameter,
both hard

hard craggy mass
fixed to skin and
deeper tissue
4 cm x 3 cm

peau d'orange

Fig. 21.4 Example of a recording of the presence of a breast mass in the medical notes. A simple diagram provides unambiguous objective information.

Axillary lymphadenopathy can be palpated only if the muscles forming the walls of the axilla are relaxed. Stand on the patient's right-hand side, support the patient's right upper arm with your right hand, and encourage the patient to allow you to take the weight of the arm (Fig. 21.5). Palpate the axilla with your left hand flat against the lateral chest wall, reaching high up into the axilla with your fingertips, sweeping around all of the walls. The left axilla is examined in a similar manner, but with the opposite hand.

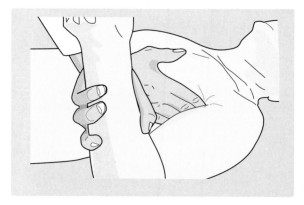

Fig. 21.5 Examination of the axilla for lymphadenopathy. It is important to support the patient's arm to relax the muscles of the axillary folds.

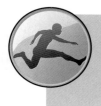 The key to successful examination of the axilla is to insure that the arm is totally relaxed and supported by your hand.

If any mass is detected in the breast or axilla, the supraclavicular and cervical lymph nodes should also be examined.

Finally, note the size of the patient's arms. Lymphedema can result from tumor invasion of the lymphatics, axillary dissection, or radiotherapy.

Breast mass

Presentation with a breast mass is common. Clearly, the most important diagnosis to exclude is carcinoma of the breast. The most common causes are listed below.

Carcinoma of the breast

In the presence of a breast mass, features that suggest carcinoma include:

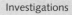

- A hard, craggy mass.
- Fixation of the mass to skin or deeper tissues.
- Nipple deviation or retraction.
- Skin changes (peau d'orange, tethering, ulceration).
- Axillary lymphadenopathy.
- Signs of systemic disease.

Fibroadenoma

A fibroadenoma is typically a well-demarcated, highly mobile, nontender mass in a young or middle-aged woman.

Fibroadenosis (cystic hyperplasia, fibrocystic disease)

The features of fibroadenosis are highly variable and depend upon the degree of cystic change, fibrosis, and masses. Often there is a diffuse change in texture in the breasts with multiple masses that are poorly defined. Mild tenderness is common.

Abscess

Abscesses usually present in lactating women and are easily distinguished by the presence of:

- Tenderness.
- Erythema.
- Poor definition.
- Axillary lymphadenopathy.
- Systemic features of infection (e.g., fever, tachycardia).

Fat necrosis

Fat necrosis is much more common in large breasts following a history of trauma. The lump is usually hard and may be tethered to the skin. It may be distinguishable from a breast carcinoma by the lack of axillary lymphadenopathy or peau d'orange.

Breast pain

The more common causes of breast pain are:

- Fibroadenosis.
- Premenstrual tension.
- Mastitis.
- Abscess.

The cause is usually apparent from the history and physical examination. Breast carcinoma rarely presents with pain.

Gynecomastia

Gynecomastia results from an increase in breast tissue. It may be unilateral or bilateral and is confirmed by palpation. The most common causes are:

- Puberty. Normal finding (very common), including in boys.
- Old age.
- Liver failure (look for stigmata of chronic liver disease).
- Carcinoma of the lung.
- Testicular tumors.
- Adrenal tumors.
- Drugs (e.g., spironolactone, cimetidine, digoxin).
- Androgen insensitivity syndrome (very rare).
- Pituitary tumors.

Investigations

The cause of many breast lesions is often apparent from a careful history and physical examination. However, in many circumstances it is important to exclude breast carcinoma. The most reliable procedure for such exclusion is to perform an excision biopsy, but it is clearly desirable to avoid this for benign lesions.

Mammography is performed as a screening procedure in the U.S. for women over 50 years of age. In the presence of a lump, mammography provides a useful adjunct by detecting areas of calcification, which are indicative of an underlying carcinoma. In addition, a second suspicious area may also be revealed, which should also be investigated clinically.

Ultrasound can be used to identify the composition (i.e., solid vs. cystic) of a mass. Cystic lesions can be aspirated as a diagnostic or therapeutic procedure. Ultrasound is often requested to localize masses before surgery. In addition, ultrasound can be used to identify masses for fine-needle aspiration (FNA). FNA may provide adequate cytological information to increase or decrease the clinical index of suspicion of malignancy, and so determine the urgency of treatment.

One last thought: men also get breast cancer, although it is rare. It also carries a worse prognosis because often the lump is already adherent to the chest wall at presentation.

187

22. Musculoskeletal Examination

Examination routine

Musculoskeletal assessment is fundamental as information on the patient's functional ability is assessed and integrated with other physical signs. Clearly, if a patient describes decreased mobility, weakness, or joint pain, a more detailed general assessment is necessary. Equally, if a focal abnormality is detected, it should be fully examined.

This chapter is not intended to provide a detailed description of examination of every joint and muscle group, but illustrates a methodical and functional approach to examining the system.

Patient exposure and position

In examining muscle groups or mobility, it is important to insure that patients are properly exposed. They should be provided with a blanket and asked to strip to their underwear in a warm, well-lit room. The initial formal assessment is usually performed on the examination table. The approach to examining a joint should follow the scheme of "look, feel, move."

 The most important part of the musculoskeletal examination is inspection.

Inspection
General inspection

Remember that the examination begins as soon as the patient walks into the examination room! It is often possible to form an impression of functional ability by observing how easily the patient gets out of the chair, walks to the examination room, and climbs onto the examination table. Note the following.

 Always try to relate pathological signs to a functional disability such as difficulty in performing routine daily activities (e.g., getting out of bed, writing, walking, picking up a knife and fork).

Age and sex
Different disease processes are more likely to occur at different ages. For example:
- Osteoarthritis and polymyalgia rheumatica are more common in the elderly.
- Osteoporosis is primarily a disease of postmenopausal women.
- Ankylosing spondylitis usually presents in young men.
- Many inflammatory arthritides first present in young women.

Racial origin
Many forms of arthritis or diseases presenting with impaired mobility have a strong genetic predisposition and are more common in certain racial groups. Others have a predominantly environmental cause that varies geographically. For example:
- Systemic lupus erythematosus (SLE) is much more common in African-American women.
- Paget's disease is more common in Caucasians.
- Multiple sclerosis is more common in patients from temperate climates.

General health and appearance
Note whether the patient appears well or is cachexic. Obesity predisposes to osteoarthritis of the back and weight-bearing joints. Cachexia may indicate chronic systemic disease or carcinoma. Note whether the patient appears to be in pain at rest or on walking. An obvious focal weakness may be apparent. These visual clues may contrast with the information obtained from the history or when the patient knows that a formal examination is being performed.

Facial appearance
Note the appearance of facial asymmetry or obvious weakness. In addition, note the general appearance (e.g., myopathic facies of muscular dystrophy with unlined expressionless facies and wasting of the facial muscles).

How easily does the patient get out of a chair?
Proximal muscle weakness (e.g., due to polymyalgia rheumatica, steroid myopathy, hyperthyroidism) will have a profound effect on getting up from a seated position. The significance of a patient wincing with pain when they rise from the chair is unclear.

Does the patient require any aids for walking?
Observe whether the patient walks unaided into the examination room, walks with the aid of a walking stick or other assistive device, or holds on to another person for support. The patient will hold a walking stick in the hand opposite the weakest leg.

    If the patient has a walker, observe how he or she uses it. It is not infrequent for a nervous but mobile patient to become reliant upon a frame. On observation the patient is seen to carry the frame in front of him/herself rather than rely upon it for support.

Gait
If the patient walks unaided, make a quick assessment of gait. A more formal assessment should be made later in the detailed examination.

How easily does the patient climb onto the examination table?
A certain amount of agility is needed for elderly patients to climb onto the examination table. It may be instructive to observe the patient during this process.

Detailed inspection
Once the patient is properly exposed and positioned, a detailed inspection should be performed. This process forms the key to a successful examination.

    A detailed examination of the musculoskeletal system is time-consuming and tiring for the patient. With the benefit of the history, a focused examination is possible after detailed inspection. The more important features to note are outlined below.

Skin rash
Skin rashes may suggest an underlying inflammatory condition:

- Infection.
- Malignancy.
- Pain.

Muscle bulk
Note the general muscle bulk and the distribution of any atrophy. For example:
- Disuse atrophy in a hemiplegic limb.
- Atrophy of the quadriceps in the presence of a proximal myopathy.
- Atrophy of the distal muscles of the lower limbs (Charcot–Marie–Tooth disease).
- Old polio.

Deformity or swelling
Observe any obvious deformity that may be the result of bone, joint, or muscle disease.
For example:
- Scoliosis.
- Varus or valgus deformity (see Fig. 22.16). This is common in the knees in osteoarthritis.
- Rigid back with loss of lumbar lordosis and fixed posture in ankylosing spondylitis.
- Obvious joint swelling. The distribution of swollen (or inflamed) joints should be mapped out as the distribution is often characteristic of the underlying disease and variations can be correlated with changes in disease activity (Fig. 22.1).

Gait
A formal assessment of the gait should be part of the routine examination, especially in an elderly patient. Apart from highlighting a possible etiological factor for impaired mobility, it provides a direct functional assessment and an impression of the problems with daily living.

    Ask the patient to walk in a straight line, turn around, and then walk back to you. Balance and ataxia may be additionally tested by asking the patient to walk heel-to-toe. Characteristic gaits may be noted as follows.

Ataxic gait
An ataxic gait is characteristically wide-based. The arms are often held out wide to aid balance. Marked clumsiness is obvious on walking heel-to-toe. The patient often staggers to the left or right. This is associated with cerebellar pathology.

Spastic gait
If the patient has spastic paraplegia, the gait is stiff and described as a "scissor gait." The appearance may resemble someone wading through water. If the

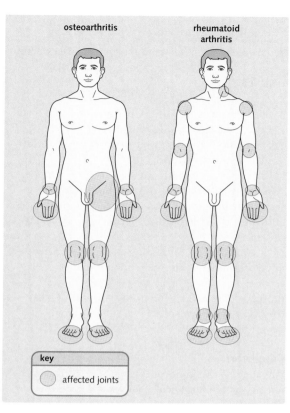

osteoarthritis   rheumatoid arthritis

key
◯ affected joints

Fig. 22.1 Typical patterns of joint involvement in two different forms of polyarthritis. In rheumatoid arthritis there is usually a symmetrical polyarthropathy. Osteoarthritis is less likely to be symmetrical but often is symmetrical in its widespread form.

patient has hemiplegia, the affected leg is extended and the leg is swung around the hip joint.

Sensory ataxia
Peripheral neuropathy with sensory ataxia results in a high-stepping gait with the appearance that the feet are being "thrown." The feet tend to be "slapped" on the floor, and the patient walks on a wide base. Romberg's test is positive (see Chapter 18). Patients often appear to be concentrating hard on where their feet are being placed.

High-stepping gait
In the presence of foot drop the affected foot is lifted high off the ground to avoid scraping the toes on the floor. Such patients are unable to stand on their heels.

Parkinsonian gait
The patient has a characteristic stooped appearance. The gait is shuffling and hesitant with short steps and a lack of associated arm movement. The arms do not usually swing during walking. The gait is described as "festinant," that is, it seems that the patient is always chasing his or her own sense of gravity. The patient often has great difficulty when asked to stop and turn around, and usually other features of Parkinson's disease are present.

Osteogenic gait
Patients with legs of unequal length may walk normally in shoes with appropriate shoelifts, but the abnormality should be obvious when they walk barefoot.

Waddling gait
A proximal myopathy is associated with a waddling gait. The patient walks on a wide base with the trunk moving from side to side on each step and the pelvis drooping as the leg leaves the ground.

Observe whether the patient has any pain on walking and, if so, which movements appear to provoke the pain.

Regional examination

The history from the patient will point you to the region of the body that needs to be examined. Specific regional examination can now begin. As with other systems of the body, it is important to follow a strict routine. When examining any region of the body or joint, use the following routine.

Inspection
Note the bones, alignment, joint swelling, redness, deformity, local swelling, and the presence of any scars.

Palpation
Palpate the area concerned, paying particular attention to:
- Skin temperature. In particular, note any areas of increased warmth. Compare the two sides.
- Tenderness. Map out any areas of tenderness and try to relate it to the affected structure.
- Deformity. Note the bony contours and any fixed flexion deformity.
- Soft tissues. Note the presence of any abnormal swellings (e.g., fluid in the joint, cysts, bursae, tumors). Palpate the muscles for bulk, etc.

Assessment of joint movement

Assess the range of active and passive movement, muscular power, and whether movement is accompanied by pain. It is important to have an appreciation of the range of normal movement around each joint. It is often helpful to test the unaffected side first so that any deviation can be more easily appreciated.

Sensation

Test the sensory modalities (see Chapter 18). Light touch, pinprick, and vibration are the most discriminatory.

Function

The most useful part of the examination is to assess the function of the relevant body part. Try to relate your assessment to daily activities. For example:

- In the lower limb, test the ability to walk, jump, hop, run.
- In the hand, test the ability to hold a pen and grip strength.

General examination

It is very important to perform a systemic examination. The localized joint symptoms may form part of a systemic disease or be referred from another site. Furthermore, it is possible to place the disability into context only when the patient is considered as a whole.

Hands

Most systemic examinations start with examination of the hands, where stigmata of systemic disease are often manifest. This is also true for a patient presenting with impaired mobility. Furthermore, many patients specifically complain of symptoms directly related to their hands (e.g., paresthesias, weakness, joint pain). A methodical approach to examination of the hands is therefore useful.

Inspection

Remember to look at the face of the patient first for any clues to the underlying disease or treatment (e.g., scleroderma, Cushingoid facies). Look at both hands. Ask the patient to place his or her hands flat on the table, palmar surface downward. Look at:

- The general shape of the hands and note any deformity (e.g., ulnar deviation in rheumatoid arthritis).

- The color of the skin (e.g., pigmentation, icterus, erythema, rash).
- The nails. Look for signs of psoriasis (e.g., pitting, onycholysis), clubbing, splinter hemorrhages, nailfold infarcts.
- Soft tissue. Note any swellings (e.g., Heberden's nodes in osteoarthritis on the proximal and distal interphalangeal joints, gouty tophi).
- Joints. Look for any swelling or redness suggestive of an active arthritis.

Ask the patient to turn his or her hands over so that the palmar aspect can be inspected. Repeat the same process of inspection. In particular, note the presence of palmar erythema, and pay close attention to the muscle bulk of the thenar eminence (atrophy in carpal tunnel syndrome) and hypothenar eminence (atrophy in T1 root lesion or in the presence of severe rheumatoid arthritis). Note the presence of any scars (e.g., carpal tunnel decompression).

Palpation

Palpate over the joints of the hand and wrist gently, noting any tenderness of the joints. Record the distribution of any tender joints (Fig. 22.2). Many forms of polyarthritis have a characteristic distribution of joint involvement. In addition, palpate for the presence of any swellings or palmar thickening (e.g., Dupuytren's contracture, trigger finger).

Movement of the joints

Assess the movement of the joints of the hand. Try to relate this to functional activity. First, test passive movement and then active movement. If the primary problem is joint disease, useful tests might include:

- Grip strength.
- Pincer grip (ask the patient to pick up a pen and write his or her name).

Assess whether movement is limited by deformity, pain, or muscular weakness. Some of the signs of rheumatoid arthritis are illustrated in Fig. 22.3.

Neurological assessment

Symptoms in the hand may result from a nerve lesion. Test sensation on the middle finger (median nerve), little finger (ulnar nerve), and the anatomical snuff box (radial nerve). The most common pathologies are:

Fig. 22.2 Patterns of joint involvement in some systemic polyarthropathies. (A) Osteoarthritis. Joint swelling of the first carpometacarpal joints is characteristic. Joint involvement is usually symmetrical in the hands and typically affects the distal interphalangeal joints. (B) Rheumatoid arthritis. Active synovitis is detected by joint warmth, swelling, redness, and tenderness. During a flare, arthritis is usually symmetrical, affecting the wrists and metacarpophalangeal and proximal interphalangeal joints. The distal interphalangeal joints are usually spared. (C) Systemic lupus erythematosus (SLE). The distribution of joint involvement is similar to that of rheumatoid arthritis in the hands, but the signs are usually less marked and pain is often out of proportion to the signs of synovitis. (D) Gout. Initial attacks of gout usually present in the lower limb, especially the first metatarsophalangeal joint. However, it may present in the hands. It is often monoarticular. The distal interphalangeal joints are more prone to attacks.

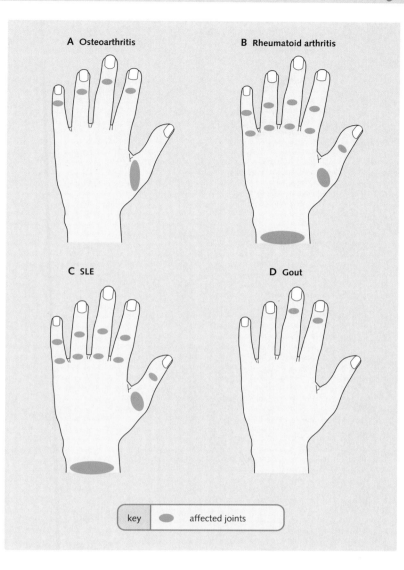

- Peripheral nerve. Radial nerve injury, most commonly at the spiral groove of the humerus, leads to wrist drop and a weak grip. The ulnar nerve is most commonly injured at the elbow, and this leads to claw hand with wasting of the muscles between the metacarpals. The medial nerve is also commonly injured at the wrist (as in carpal tunnel syndrome), and this leads to wasting of the thenar eminence.
- Nerve root or brachial plexus lesion (e.g., Pancoast's tumor).
- Sensory neuropathy.

When examining motor and sensory function, consider the implication of each elicited physical sign and whether the underlying problem is likely to be nerve root, peripheral nerve, muscular, or joint pathology.

Motor function tests

The tests of motor function are illustrated in Fig. 22.4. If the problem is unilateral, it is very helpful to directly compare strength in the two hands, testing the normal hand first.

193

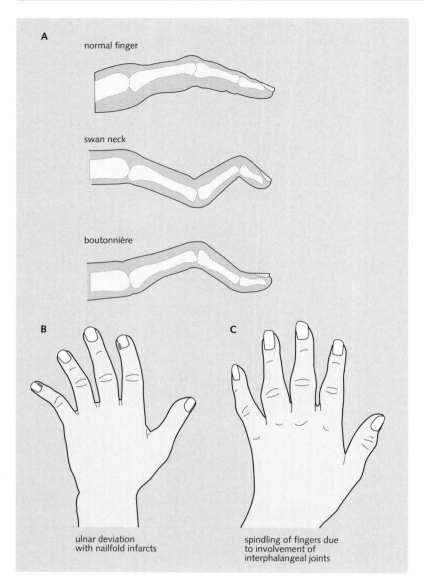

A normal finger

swan neck

boutonnière

B ulnar deviation with nailfold infarcts

C spindling of fingers due to involvement of interphalangeal joints

Fig. 22.3 Signs of rheumatoid arthritis in the hands. (A) Deformities of the fingers result from tendon rupture and joint laxity. Characteristic patterns include swan neck and boutonnière deformities. (B) Ulnar deviation results from subluxation at the metacarpophalangeal joints. Nailfold infarcts are one of the manifestations of vasculitis. (C) Spindling of the fingers is an early sign due to involvement and swelling of the interphalangeal joints.

Sensory function tests

Test sensory function in the hand, including the different modalities (pinprick, light touch, vibration, and joint position). The distribution of sensory loss is illustrated for the three peripheral nerves as well as the dermatomes in Fig. 22.5. Remember that the areas of skin providing sensory fibers for the peripheral nerves or nerve roots often overlap, so it is important to test in the more discriminating areas.

Clues from the systemic examination

It should be apparent from the history and assessment of the hands whether the lesion is articular, vascular, neurological, etc. There are often clues to be obtained from a systemic survey. For example:
- Look at the elbows for rheumatoid nodules or a psoriatic rash.
- Note the presence of gouty tophi on the ear lobes.

Fig. 22.4 Movements of (A) the fingers and (B) the thumb. Finger abduction and adduction (e.g., "Grip a piece of paper between your fingers") rely on the ulnar nerve. Thumb extension relies on the radial nerve; opposition, flexion, and abduction rely on the median nerve.

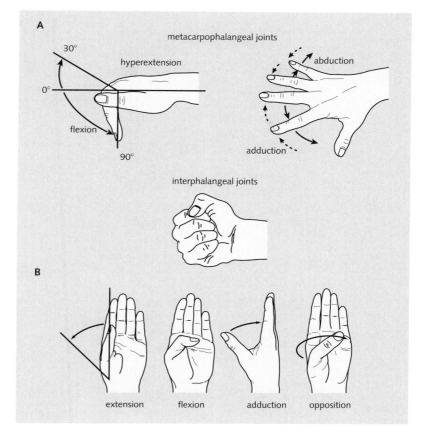

- If the patient has an arthritis, it is essential to examine each joint so that the distribution of joint involvement can be mapped out.

Shoulder examination

The shoulder is a difficult joint to examine because it moves in so many different ways! Expose the patient. Ask him/her to strip to the waist and sit on the end of the table.

Look

Inspect the patient for any signs of skin erythema or scars. Note any asymmetry between the two shoulders. Look for evidence of wasting of the deltoid muscles and effusions or joint swelling. Observe the position of the shoulders.

Feel

Palpate over all the joints that encompass the shoulder: the sternoclavicular joints, the acromioclavicular joints, and the glenohumeral joints. Pay attention to any joint line tenderness or swelling.

Move

First, ask the patient to do the moving (active movement). Ask the patient to move the shoulder through abduction, flexion, extension, and internal and external rotation (Fig 22.6). A good way to do this is to ask patients to place their hand behind their neck and slide their hand downward between their shoulders.

Second, you should move the shoulder through a full range of movement (passive movement) and see how far you can move the shoulder before the patient experiences pain. You should have a hand over the joint, feeling for crepitus or restrictions to movement.

Then test the power of the patient's shoulder against resistance.

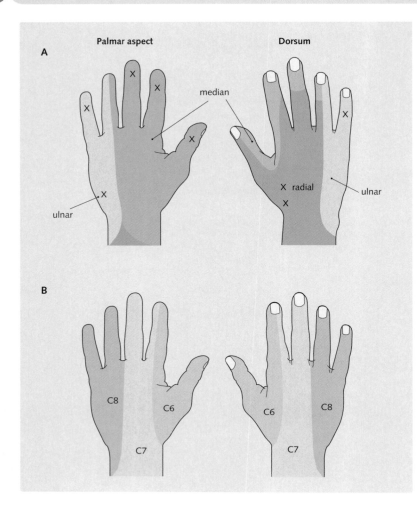

A

Palmar aspect

X
X
X

median

X

X
ulnar

ulnar

Dorsum

X

X radial
X

ulnar

B

C8
C6

C7

C6
C8

C7

Fig. 22.5 (A) Dermatomes corresponding to the peripheral nerve supply of the hand. The crosses indicate the more useful places for assessing sensation in a quick examination. (B) Dermatomes corresponding to the nerve root supply.

Examining the glenohumeral joint

Immobilize the scapula by placing a hand on it to restrain it. Ask patients to abduct their arm (which must start down by their side). If they cannot initiate this movement, there is probably a rotator cuff tear. If abduction is restricted and further passive movement causes more pain, this is classed as "impingement pain." The patient is likely to have painful arc syndrome.

The rotator cuff consists of the supraspinatus, subscapularis, and infraspinatus tendons. An incomplete tear leads to painful arc syndrome (pain on movement from 45–140°). A complete tear results in the inability to initiate abduction. If you abduct the patient's arm to greater than 45°, the patient should be able to continue the abduction to 180°.

Elbow
Look

Expose the patient to the waist and inspect both elbows from behind with the arms in extension. Look for any obvious deformity. Is there an effusion filling out the hollow at the head of the radius?

Feel

Palpate the bony contours of the elbow. Palpate over the epicondyles and radial head. Feel for any signs of inflammation or bursae.

Move

The elbow should move freely from 0 to 150° (normal people also get a little extension). While doing this, palpate over the elbow joint and the head of the radius, feeling for crepitus.

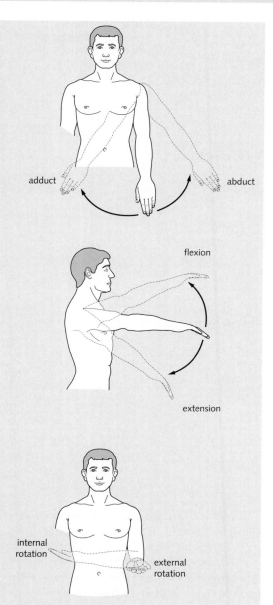

adduct — abduct

flexion

extension

internal rotation — external rotation

Fig. 22.6 Shoulder movements.

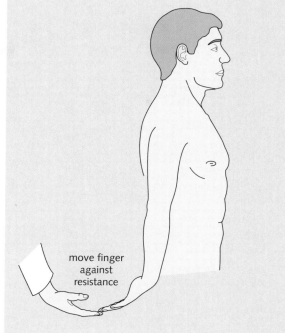

move finger against resistance

Fig. 22.7 Golfer's elbow. If moving the fingers against resistance causes pain, then the patient has golfer's elbow.

flex the elbow and squeeze your hand. If the patient has tennis elbow, the second maneuver should be less painful. Figure 22.7 shows how to test for golfer's elbow (medial epicondylitis). Affected patients are tender over the respective epicondyles.

Back

Back pain is a very common presentation, both to primary care practitioners and hospital doctors. It is necessary to develop a systematic approach for examining patients with back pain so that potentially serious disease can be recognized early and investigated, while appropriate advice can be offered to the vast majority with less serious but nonetheless disabling problems.

Now fix the elbow at the patient's side and flex the arm to 90°. Test pronation and supination. With the elbow fully extended, test the integrity of the collateral ligaments.

To test for tennis elbow (lateral epicondylitis), ask the patient to fully extend the elbow and then to squeeze your hand. Then ask the patient to slightly

In the context of back pain, neurological examination of the legs is important. Spinal cord compression warrants urgent investigation.

197

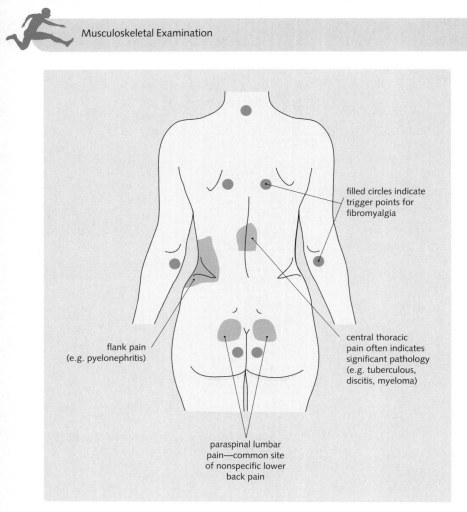

Fig. 22.8 The site of back tenderness is important because it may correspond to the etiology.

filled circles indicate trigger points for fibromyalgia

central thoracic pain often indicates significant pathology (e.g. tuberculous, discitis, myeloma)

flank pain (e.g. pyelonephritis)

paraspinal lumbar pain—common site of nonspecific lower back pain

Inspection

A brief survey of the patient often provides invaluable clues. In particular, note:

- General health (e.g., cachexia suggestive of underlying malignancy).
- Posture and deformity (e.g., kyphosis, scoliosis, loss of lumbar lordosis).
- Scars (e.g., previous surgery to the back).
- Pain. Note whether the patient appears to be in pain and is lying very still for fear of provoking worse pain, whether the patient is comfortable at rest, and whether or not the patient is pain-free on moving around.

Examination of the back

Palpate the back for local tenderness suggestive of an inflammatory process. Record in the notes the site of elicited tenderness. This may indicate the underlying disease (Fig. 22.8).

Examine the movements involving the vertebrae (flexion, extension, lateral flexion, rotation) and record both the range of movement and any pain elicited (Fig. 22.9). If ankylosing spondylitis is suspected, the sacroiliac joints must be assessed because they are often the first site of inflammation. Lateral compression of the pelvis may elicit pain in the presence of sacroiliitis.

Peripheral joints and systemic examination for arthritis

A full survey of other joints may reveal a more widespread arthropathy (e.g., ankylosing spondylitis, psoriatic arthropathy). Note the distribution of joint involvement and the presence of active synovitis.

In addition, there may also be nonarticular clues to the presence of a systemic arthritis. For example:

- Psoriatic arthropathy is associated with a classic rash and nail changes.

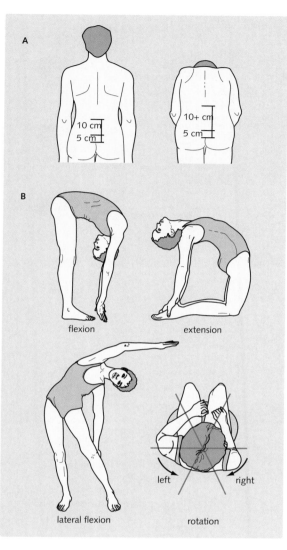

Fig. 22.9 Assessing movements of the (A) lumbar and (B) thoracic spine. Flexion of the lumbar spine can be objectively measured. Ask patients to touch their toes, keeping their knees straight. Mark the spine at the lumbosacral junction 5 cm and 10 cm above this point. The distance between the upper two points should move approximately 5 cm on full flexion. This movement is impaired in ankylosing spondylitis.

- Ankylosing spondylitis is associated with decreased chest expansion, upper lobe fibrosis, iritis, and aortic regurgitation.

Test for evidence of nerve root entrapment
Acute or chronic back pain may be due to a prolapsed intervertebral disk, which may be associated with sciatic nerve root entrapment. The presence of nerve root entrapment and its localization may be elicited by testing:
- Straight leg raising.
- Femoral stretch test (Fig. 22.10).

Neurological examination of the legs
It is important to exclude nerve root pressure or spinal cord compression. A description of the neurological assessment of the legs is given in Chapter 18.

Detailed systemic examination
A detailed systemic examination should always be performed in a patient presenting with new-onset or progressive back pain. The back pain may be a manifestation of a systemic disease (e.g., metastatic carcinoma) or be referred from a source in the abdomen or pelvis. For example:
- Chronic pancreatitis.
- Carcinoma of the pancreas.
- Posterior duodenal ulcer.
- Aortic aneurysm.
- Retroperitoneal fibrosis.

Hips
The hip is a common site of osteoarthritis in the elderly, but pathology sometimes begins in infancy or childhood. It is important to recognize disease early in its natural history so that appropriate treatment can be instituted.

The initial part of the examination is performed with the patient lying flat and properly exposed. Later, posture and gait can be formally assessed.

Position
Start by insuring that the pelvis is set square so that leg length and deformity can be assessed accurately (Fig. 22.11). Attempt to position the line joining the anterior superior iliac spines perpendicular to the legs. If this is not possible, there is a fixed abduction or adduction deformity.

Inspection
Note the presence of any scars (e.g., previous hip replacement), abnormal bony or soft tissue contours, and any abnormalities of the skin (e.g., erythema, sinuses).

Palpation
Palpate for any tenderness or warmth.

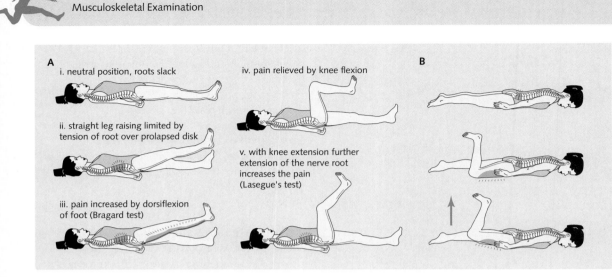

A

i. neutral position, roots slack

ii. straight leg raising limited by tension of root over prolapsed disk

iii. pain increased by dorsiflexion of foot (Bragard test)

iv. pain relieved by knee flexion

v. with knee extension further extension of the nerve root increases the pain (Lasegue's test)

B

Fig. 22.10 Stretch tests. (A) Straight leg raising. Record the angle (normally 80–90°) through which each leg can be raised. (B) Femoral stretch test.

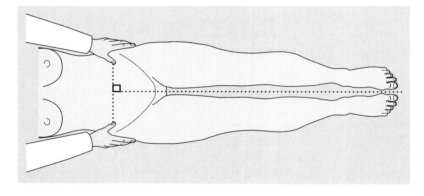

Fig. 22.11 Setting the pelvis square. Ask the patient to lie flat upon the examination table. Palpate the anterior superior iliac spines. Move the pelvis so that they are square to the lower limbs.

Measurement of leg length

If the pelvis is square, it is easy to estimate relative leg length by inspection. However, if there is any doubt, the leg can be measured from the anterior superior iliac spine to the medial malleolus (Fig. 22.12). An apparent discrepancy can be excluded by measuring the distance from the xiphisternum to the medial malleolus.

Examination for fixed deformity

Longstanding arthritis commonly results in a contracture of the joint capsule or muscles and subsequent fixed flexion deformity. Often patients compensate by increasing their lumbar lordosis (Fig. 22.13). This may be assessed by placing a hand behind the lumbar spine to detect a lordosis and then asking patients to fully flex their good leg. Push the leg further into flexion to obliterate the lordosis and observe the angle of fixed flexion deformity in the affected hip.

Assessment of movements about the hip

It is important to assess movement about the hip and to eliminate movement of the pelvis that may compensate for deficiencies. Assess the range of movement for passive and active movements. The normal range of movement is illustrated in Fig. 22.14.

Active movement should also be tested to assess power using the Medical Research Council (MRC) grading of strength (see Fig. 18.11).

Fig. 22.12 Assessing relative leg length. (A) Measure from the anterior superior iliac spine to just below the medial malleolus on each side. (B) If the pelvis is tilted, the leg length may appear discrepant. (C) Apparent shortening may be detected by measuring the distance from the xiphisternum to the medial malleolus.

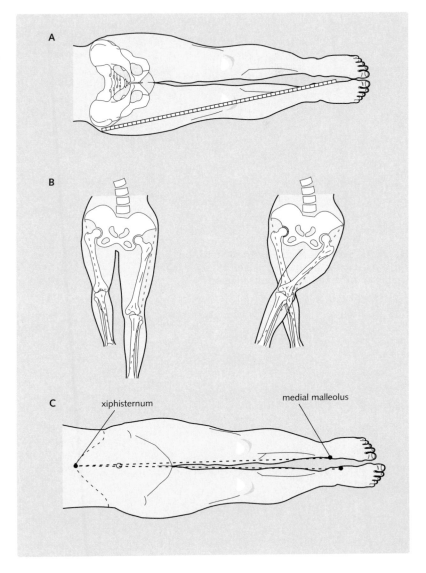

Gait and posture

Ask the patient to stand up. The Trendelenburg test should be performed to assess the postural stability of the hip joint (particularly the gluteal muscles). Normally, if one leg is lifted off the ground, the abductors will stabilize the leg and the pelvis will tilt up on the side of the lifted leg. If the abductors are ineffective, the body weight is too much for the adductors and the hip will tilt downwards (Fig. 22.15).

The causes of a positive Trendelenburg test are:
- Paralysis of the abductor muscles (e.g., polio).
- Absence of stability (e.g., ununited fracture of the femoral neck).

Finally, assess the gait.

Systemic survey

Remember to perform a systemic survey for other causes of hip symptoms.

Knee
Inspection

With the patient properly exposed and supine on a table, inspect the knee, thigh, and lower leg, noting:

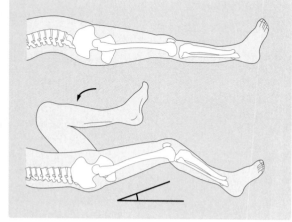

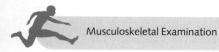

Fig. 22.13 Examination for fixed flexion deformity of the hip. A fixed deformity may be hidden by increasing the lumbar lordosis. This should be eliminated.

Normal range of movement at the hip joint	
Movement	**Range (degrees)**
flexion	0–120
extension	0 (extension occurs by rotating the pelvis)
abduction	0–30
adduction	0–30
lateral rotation	40
medial rotation	40

Fig. 22.14 Normal range of movement at the hip joint.

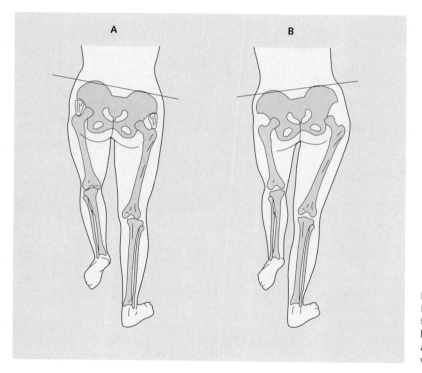

Fig. 22.15 Trendelenburg test. (A) Normally the hip abductors will tilt the pelvis upward when the leg is lifted off the ground. (B) If the abductors cannot sustain the weight, the pelvis will droop.

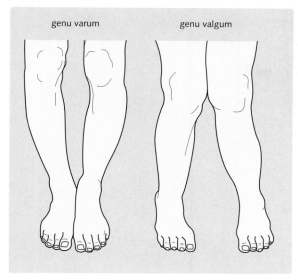

genu varum   genu valgum

Fig. 22.16 Genu varum and genu valgum.

- Muscle bulk and evidence of wasting.
- Bony deformity (e.g., genu varum, genu valgum, Fig. 22.16).
- Evidence of soft tissue swelling or effusion.

Palpation

Palpate the bony contours of the knee joint noting any areas of tenderness or warmth. Specifically examine for an effusion. A small effusion may only be detectable by massaging fluid into the suprapatellar pouch and observing accumulation in the medial compartment by pressure over the superior and lateral aspects of the joint. A larger effusion is detectable by the patellar tap.

Movements

Assess for the presence of a fixed flexion deformity, the range of passive movement, and strength of active movement.

Tests of stability

The four major ligaments should be tested in turn as follows:

- Medial and lateral ligaments (Fig. 22.17A). Support the knee in a position close to full extension and ask patients to relax their muscles. Apply an abduction and adduction force in turn to test the integrity of the medial and lateral ligaments respectively.
- Anterior and posterior cruciate ligaments (Fig. 22.17B). The anterior cruciate ligament prevents anterior displacement of the tibia on the femur. The posterior cruciate prevents posterior displacement. Flex the knee and fix the foot firmly on the table by sitting lightly on it. Clasp the knee joint with both hands, holding your fingers behind the joint and thumbs laterally so that the tips are resting on each femoral condyle. Alternately push and pull the tibia to assess anteroposterior stability.

Fig. 22.17 Testing for stability of the knee joint. (A) Medial and lateral collateral ligaments. (B) Cruciate ligaments.

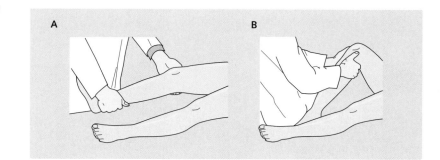

A   B

Overview

Ophthalmic examination is essential in any detailed assessment of a patient. Not only may the cause of visual symptoms be determined, but the retina is the only place where the small blood vessels of the body can be directly visualized, providing clues to a host of systemic diseases.

Examination routine

Inspection

Before fundoscopy, look at the eyes for:
- Red eye (e.g., conjunctivitis, iritis, acute glaucoma, scleritis).
- Pupil size, symmetry, and irregularity.
- Pupil reflexes.
- Arcus senilis (significant in young adults).
- Squint.
- Ptosis.

Visual acuity

Test near and distant vision. Visual acuity should be tested in any complete physical examination. Test each eye individually with patients wearing their own glasses or contact lenses to correct any refractive error. This need take only a few seconds and can be adapted to different circumstances. For example:
- Read a newspaper headline from the other side of the room.
- Count fingers from the end of the bed.
- Identify light from dark, perceive hand movements.

If time permits, perform a formal assessment with a Snellen chart (Fig. 23.1). The patient should be placed 20 feet from a standard chart and asked to read the letters. The last line that can be clearly distinguished by the patient should be recorded for each eye. Accepted normal vision is 20/20. The denominator refers to the distance from the chart that an normal eye can read what the person being tested can read at 20 feet. Near vision can be formally tested with special books with text of a defined font and pitch size.

Eye movements and nystagmus

These are discussed in Chapter 18. Squint may be assessed by the cover test. If the eye fixating an object is covered, the squinting eye will move to take up fixation.

Fundoscopy

Examine in a darkened room to maximize pupil size. Ophthalmologists and diabetologists will dilate the pupil if there is no contraindication. The patient should look straight ahead and focus on the far wall. First set the ophthalmoscope so that you can see through it in an undistorted manner (especially if you normally wear glasses). Familiarize yourself with the way a fundoscope works.

Practice fundoscopy on as many normal people as possible. It will become easier to recognize any pathological signs.

Red reflex

Start by shining the light from about 12 inches on the pupil to look for a red reflex. Loss of red reflex is usually due to vitreous hemorrhage or a dense cataract. Bring the ophthalmoscope closer to the eye and focus on the retina, looking systematically at the following.

Anterior chamber

Using a +10 lens, focus on the iris and examine for rubeosis, hypopyon, etc. Then by decreasing the power of the ophthalmoscope, focus through the anterior chamber, lens, and posterior chamber. Small cataracts appear black and well demarcated using this technique.

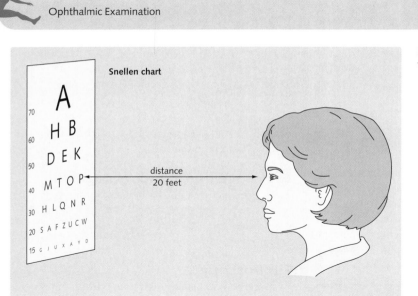

Fig. 23.1 Use of Snellen chart to test visual acuity.

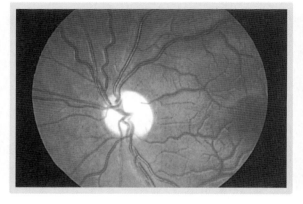

Fig. 23.2 Optic atrophy. (Courtesy of Myron Yanoff.)

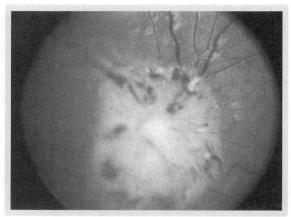

Fig. 23.3 Papilledema (swelling of the optic disk) caused by acute lymphoplastic leukemia. (Courtesy of Myron Yanoff.)

Optic disk

Note the size of the disk and color. The most important pathologies to note are:

- Optic atrophy (Fig. 23.2) may be due to multiple sclerosis, compression of the optic nerve (e.g., by pituitary tumor, aneurysm).
- Papilledema (Fig. 23.3) may be due to accelerated hypertension, a space-occupying lesion, hydrocephalus, benign intracranial hypertension (especially in obese women), cavernous sinus thrombosis, central retinal vein thrombosis.
- Glaucoma: pathological cupping of the disk due to gradual loss of nerve fibers and supporting glial cells, resulting in a pale disk with an enlarged cup.
- Myelinated nerve fibers.

Retina

Note the retinal vessels. Trace the vessels away from the optic disk toward each quadrant of the retina in turn. Alternatively, you can trace a vessel centrally from the periphery to the optic disk. The veins are darker and appear wider than the arteries. The main features to observe about the retinal vessels are:

- Engorgement of the veins, which implies slow flow (e.g., retinal venous occlusion, polycythemia).
- Attenuation of the arterioles (e.g., due to retinal artery occlusion, widespread retinal atrophy).
- Arteriovenous (AV) nicking in hypertension.

206

Note the retinal background in each quadrant. In particular, look for:

- Hemorrhages. The most common hemorrhages are flame-shaped hemorrhages, which are superficial and occur in severe hypertension. "Dot hemorrhages" are not true bleeding areas but represent microaneurysms, which are prone to rupture, forming "blot" hemorrhages.
- Hard exudates (true retinal exudates). These are usually small, sharply defined, and intensely white.
- Soft exudates (areas of infarction). These have a fluffy appearance resembling cotton wool. They usually have an ill-defined edge.
- Neovascularization. New blood vessel formation is an important sign of diabetic retinopathy. These new blood vessels are fragile and appear as a tuft of delicate vessels on the surface of the retina.
- Photocoagulation scars.
- Pigmentation (retinitis pigmentosa).

Some of the more important fundal abnormalities are illustrated in Figs. 23.4 and 23.5.

Diabetic patients should have detailed fundoscopy at least once a year. Fundal changes are sensitive markers of end-organ damage in diabetes mellitus and hypertension.

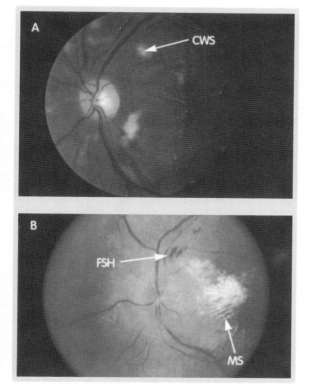

C	Features of hypertensive retinopathy
Grade I	silver wiring of arterioles
Grade II	AV nipping
Grade III	soft exudates (due to small infarcts); flame-shaped hemorrhages
Grade IV	papilledema

Fig. 23.4 (A, B) Grade III hypertension. CWS, cotton wool spot; FSH, flame-shaped hemorrhage; MS, macular star. (C) Features of hypertensive retinopathy. Grades III and IV indicate accelerated hypertension. (Courtesy of Myron Yanoff.)

207

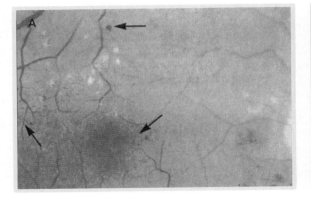

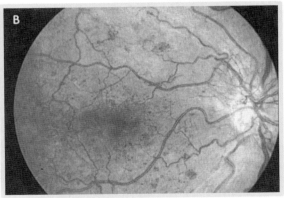

C	Features of diabetic retinopathy

background diabetic retinopathy
    dot hemorrhages (microaneurysms)
    blot hemorrhages (discrete bleed)
    hard exudates

proliferative retinopathy
    neovascularization
    (laser coagulation scars)

Fig. 23.5 Diabetic retinopathy. (A) Background changes. Arrows indicate hemorrhages. (B) Neovascularization at the optic disk. (C) Features of diabetic retinopathy. (A, B courtesy of Myron Yanoff.)

Macula

Ask the patient to look briefly directly at the light of the ophthalmoscope. Macular disease is common in the elderly.

Visual fields

The examination routine for testing by confrontation is discussed in Chapter 18. More formal visual field testing can be performed by assessing the visual threshold in different regions, but this relies upon special equipment and skilled interpretation.

24. Writing Medical Notes

General points

In writing up the medical notes, it is extremely important to adopt a systematic and objective style. Your notes form a permanent record of your impression of the patient at that moment in time. It should be possible for another healthcare professional to read your notes and to understand them and your conclusions. Although the following points appear to be obvious, it is alarming how often simple good clinical practice is ignored. Always insure that:

- Each piece of paper has the patient's name at its head. Notes have an uncanny knack of falling apart!
- Each entry is dated, and ideally a time is recorded.
- Each entry is followed by a legible signature and your name. Scrawled initials are inadequate. Someone else has to read your notes and be able to identify who has written them.
- Your handwriting is legible. This point sounds ludicrously obvious, but unfortunately anyone who has looked through a set of notes will testify that it is often forgotten.

Your handwriting must be clear and legible. It is dangerous to write illegibly!

- Each statement is objective. It is no longer acceptable to write value judgments in the notes if they cannot be justified.

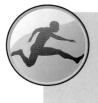

Remember that patients (or their lawyers) may gain access to the notes. Avoid the use of statements that you cannot justify.

- You write in the notes every time you see the patient. You do not have to write an essay—a short statement of the patient's progress is an important record. Even noting a lack of any change since your last visit is important.
- You avoid the use of abbreviations as much as possible. If they have to be used, use only accepted terms such as MI (myocardial infarction), LVF (left ventricular failure). Check to see if the hospital has a list of common abbreviations.
- You use diagrams where appropriate as they are often much more descriptive than long paragraphs.
- You keep your record as concise as possible.

Often the history given by the patient is recounted in an unconventional manner. When writing your notes, it is usual practice to record the history in the order described in Part I of this book. This helps to structure your own thoughts as well as those of anyone who subsequently reads the notes. There is an example of this in the chapter. Clearly the history is a dynamic process, and there are infinite variations and exceptions to this general aim.

Finally, it is important to make a note of what information has been given to the patient. Poor communication between the doctor and patient is responsible for the vast majority of instances of patient dissatisfaction, complaints, and litigation. It is helpful, not only to yourself but also for other doctors, to be aware of exactly what information the patient has when starting the next visit.

Structuring your thoughts

When you first start to take medical histories, it is a struggle to remember the traditional order of questions to ask and the normal examination routine. However, your job has only just begun! Remember that the aim of a medical examination is to:

- Identify any problems.
- Formulate a differential diagnosis of these problems.

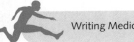

- Consider a plan of initial investigations to elucidate the underlying cause, severity, and prognosis of each problem.
- Initiate treatment and advice for the patient.

> In an examination setting, it is important to spend time reflecting on the significant points of the history and examination. Always allow enough time to gather your thoughts before presenting your findings.

Problem-oriented medical record (POMR)

The POMR is a method to document your findings. There are different formats, including the complete database write-up, which is often used for a first visit to the clinic or admission note to the hospital, and progress notes, which are often written in the SOAP (Subjective, Objective, Assessment, and Plan) format. It is often stated: "If it isn't documented in the chart, it didn't happen."

The database (history and physical exam plus)

A database for a "work-up" of a new patient is defined at the level of thoroughness desired or made necessary by time and practice circumstances.

- Patient profile: identify the patient.
- Chief complaint: why did the patient seek medical attention?
- History of the present illness (problems documented, using the Sacred 7): may be recorded chronologically in narrative fashion. Alternatively each important problem may be discussed separately and organized under the headings (Subj.–Obj.–Sig.–Negs.–Prior Rx). A third method is to discuss the primary or new problem narratively and organize a review of secondary problems as outlined above.
- Past medical history.
- Family history.
- Social history.
- High-risk behaviors history.
- Review of systems.

- Physical examination.
- Objective data (e.g., stool for occult blood, PPD skin tests, blood counts).

Different specialties may have augmented databases. For example, a cardiologist may require a much more detailed cardiac history or special cardiac examination or studies for all of his patients; thus his/her database would be different from that of a primary care physician. Figure 24.1 gives a general outline of the traditional write-up. Figure 24.2 points out common errors in student write-ups.

The database is a dynamic and changing body of clinical information. Progress notes expand the information contained in the database under the headings Subjective (S) and Objective (O).

The problem list

After finishing the complete history and physical examination, it is important to develop a problem list. It is the problem list that facilitates your development of a differential diagnosis and the ordering of tests (e.g., laboratory tests, imaging). The problem list is the first information in the chart. Its purposes include to:

- Serve as a table of contents to the patient's medical history.
- Serve as a constant reminder of all identified problems.
- Summarize the course of the medical history at a glance.
- Provide the ideal site for warning notices (e.g., allergies, drug reactions).
- Serve as a tool for provider communication.
- Serve as a health maintenance indicator.
- Provide a source for practice statistics and demography.
- Facilitate professional audits.
- Provide an index to hospital chart or office file information.

A Medical Center Problem List template is displayed in Fig. 24.3.

Definition: what is a problem?

Any identifiable factor that may have a significant influence on a patient's health and quality of life is entered on the problem list. A problem is more than a "medical" abnormality and may include those items, past and present, solved and unresolved, of major medical, psychological, social, or economic

Write-up outline

A. Database

For the patient being evaluated for the first time, the medical history may be taken in a conventional fashion and recorded in a narrative-chronological manner. You must include the history of the present illness, past medical history, social and family history, high-risk behavior history, and a review of systems. The database that has been accumulated (history, physical examination, and laboratory data) is then used to identify problems.

B. Problem list

Any identifiable factor that has or may have a significant influence on a patient's health and quality of life is entered on the problem list. A problem is more than a "medical" abnormality and may include those items, past and present, resolved and unresolved, of major medical, psychological, social, or economic significance:

A proven diagnosis—e.g., rheumatoid arthritis
A physiological entity or syndrome—e.g., congestive heart failure
A symptom—e.g., chest pain
A physical abnormality—e.g., hepatomegaly
An abnormal lab value—e.g., elevated alkaline phosphatase
A risk factor—e.g., cigarette abuse
An operation—e.g., subtotal gastrectomy
A psychological or social problem—e.g., unemployment or "cannot care for self"

C. Assessment (*"What I Think"*)

After recording the complete database and establishing the problem list, the physician considers each problem that requires clarification and/or solution and makes an assessment. This part of the record requires the physician to use his analytical sense in commencing the patient's work-up, in the same way as it will be utilized in subsequent problem-oriented progress notes. Under discussion or assessment, he/she may wish to record his/her differential diagnostic probabilities as well as to interrelate a particular problem with others. An assessment must reflect your clinical reasoning and can never be a simple differential diagnosis or a list of "rule-outs." For each problem you then write a precise plan using the following outline.

D. Plans (*"What I'm Going to Do"*)

1. **Dx**: This section lists the additional diagnostic maneuvers that are needed, such as laboratory tests, imaging procedures, and physiological monitoring.
2. **Rx**: The medications and therapeutic procedures that will be employed are listed here (e.g., abdominal paracentesis).
3. **Pt. Ed. (patient education)**: A brief statement of what the patient has been taught or is to be told about his illness is made here, e.g., "to Diabetic Clinic for instruction in insulin administration." Proper patient education is vital to comprehensive patient care; therefore, the entries made in this section are of great importance.

Fig. 24.1 Summary of write-up guidelines.

significance. On the other hand, a problem is *never* a diagnostic possibility or a "rule out." It is recorded as precisely as possible with the information available at the time of its recording. In other words, a problem may be as follows:

- A proven diagnosis (e.g., rheumatoid arthritis).
- A physiological entity or syndrome (e.g., congestive heart failure).
- A symptom (e.g., chest pain).
- A physical abnormality (e.g., hepatomegaly).
- An abnormal lab value (e.g., elevated alkaline phosphatase).
- A risk factor (e.g., cigarette abuse).
- An operation (e.g., subtotal gastrectomy).
- A psychological or social problem (e.g., unemployment or "cannot care for self").

It should be numbered as to problem and dated as to entry and onset of the problem.

Organization of the problem list

Each problem should be numbered and dated as to time of entry and time of onset. After the initial problem list is created, new problems will arise as the patient is further investigated and followed in a continuing program. Each new problem is dated and recorded under a new number on the problem list. It is necessary, however, that adequate documentation is made in the record to substantiate the problem. Each problem added to the problem list should have in the progress note section a dated note, including the number, title, and SOAP format.

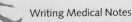

Common errors in student write-ups

1. Chief complaint
  (a) Too long
  (b) Contains symptoms which should be in present illness
  (c) Duration of complaint not mentioned

2. Present illness
  (a) Story not chronologically developed
  (b) Cannot tell whether disease is constant, remittent, or progressive
  (c) Pertinent (significant) negatives are lacking
  (d) Information not related to the problem is included

3. Systems review
  (a) Entire systems may be omitted
  (b) Specific important symptoms not mentioned
  (c) Vague generalizations about a system, e.g., "cardiovascular—negative," "pulmonary—unremarkable"

4. Patient profiles   (a) Too rigid and brief, not enough information about patient as a person
5. Past medical history   (a) Failure to elaborate on the details of important diseases such as diabetes or hypertension

6. Errors in writing
  (a) Incorrect spelling, bad grammar, poor sentence structure
  (b) Improper use of abbreviations
  (c) The frequent use of "Patient denies…, admits to…, complains of…"
  (d) Inappropriate use of scientific terms

7. Errors in problem list
  (a) Too short—omits coexisting problems
  (b) Too long—lists all symptoms and signs with no attempt to cluster clues into cohesive groups
  (c) Use of "possible," "probable," or "rule out" on the problem list. (These belong in the assessment.)

8. Physical examination
  (a) Entire system or body part not examined
  (b) Assessments given instead of description, e.g., "basal cell carcinoma" instead of "5 mm raised nodule with pearly, rolled border"
  (c) Vague terminology, e.g., "Heart—unremarkable," "Chest—normal." These are acceptable in an oral presentation but not in a write-up at this time.

9. Assessment
  (a) Failure to list all the clues that lead to labeling a problem
  (b) Not listing problems in terms of urgency and importance
  (c) Merely listing a diagnosis without providing in writing the thinking that led to decision making

10. Plan
  (a) Ordering excessive and unnecessary diagnostic procedures
  (b) Treatment plans—sometimes impracticable, ineffective, or too costly
  (c) Failure to deal with all the problems on the problem list

Fig. 24.2 Common errors in student write-ups.

Revision of the problem list

The revisions should reflect the dynamic and continuing flow of the medical record. When several problems turn out to be separate manifestations of a single problem, these problems should be grouped together using the number of the first recorded manifestation. Alternatively, one may indicate that all manifestations have been resolved to a single problem, which is given a new number. In this instance, all previous numbers are permanently dropped. Thus, "pericarditis," "arthritis," "pleural effusion," and "thrombocytopenia," originally listed as separate problems, may after further study turn out to be manifestations of "disseminated

212

MEDICAL CENTER
Tucson, Arizona

PROBLEM LIST

LOCATION _____ DATE _____

PATIENT NAME _____

PATIENT NUMBER _____

Problem No.	Onset Date	Problem	Entry Date	Problem Status/ Admit Dates	Currently Responsible Physician	Admit Notice*

Primary Care Physician	Telephone	Date
Address		
Referring Physician	Telephone	Date
Address		

UH 1-12-03 R179   *Please notify the currently responsible physician(s) of patient's admission, and enter the date notified.*

Fig. 24.3 A Medical Center Problem List template.

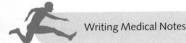

lupus." One could then use the problem heading as follows:

1. Problem No. __ Disseminated lupus.
    a. Arthritis.
    b. Pericarditis.
    c. Pleural effusion.
    d. Thrombocytopenia.

As problems are clarified, altered, further delineated, or solved, this action may be indicated by inserting an arrow after the problem. The date of change is also recorded. The purpose of this is to indicate activity and problem solution. Thus, at a glance, one can always note when problems will require further evaluation, since there will be an arrow after the problem but no indication of solution. As an example:

2. Problem No. __ Chest Pain → ASHD with infarction

The assessment (what you think) and plan (what you are going to do)

This is where the impressions of the physician are stated: "On the basis of the available data I believe the diagnosis is _____." Impressions should be backed by generally accepted reference, i.e., a general medical text. Under discussion or assessment, the clinician may wish to record his/her differential diagnostic probabilities as well as to interrelate a particular problem with others. For each problem the clinician then writes a precise plan using the following outline:

- Diagnostic (Dx). This is where additional studies are recommended and where the differential diagnosis is placed. Rule out another diagnosis by getting the following studies [list studies].
- Treatment (Rx). The medications and therapeutic procedures that will be employed are listed here.
- Patient education (Pt. Ed.) The patient is informed of coming studies, procedures, possible complications, prognosis, options, and other relevant information. This is the best "informed consent" possible.

Progress notes

Progress notes may either be in a SOAP format or a flowsheet. They are used for ongoing entries in a patient's hospital chart or to record visits to the outpatient office.

SOAP note
Organization

- S: new or important subjective information or a description of the patient's visit to the office (Sacred 7).
- O: new or important objective information about the physical examination and results of diagnostic studies.
- A: changes in the assessment, synthesis of data, or a discussion of what you think is occurring.
- P: new or changing plans or the plans related to the current problem. You should include Dx (e.g., consultation requests, biopsies, lab studies, preparation of a flowsheet to monitor progress, repeat physical examination, etc.), Rx (therapeutic interventions), and Pt. Ed. (patient education).

General points

- Each entry should be numbered and titled.
- Separate SOAP notes should made for each problem.
- Each person entering notes should identify himself: John Jones M.D., Tim Smith M.S.-3, etc.
- Always include a legible signature and a date; include a time if important.
- Redundancy does not add useful information. If someone else has already said it, don't repeat it. Good charts are not measured by weight.

Prescription writing

There are many potential pitfalls in writing prescriptions. Most are related to use of abbreviations or legibility of handwriting. You will be writing prescriptions during the majority of your career. Here are some introductory guidelines.

Abbreviations used in writing prescriptions are listed in Fig. 24.4.

Inpatient medication order

Information that needs to be included in an inpatient medication order are:

- Name of the drug.
- Dosage.
- Instructions for dispensing (Sig:).
- Route of administration.
- Dosing frequency.

Abbreviations	
Abbreviation	**Meaning**
QD, qd, qD	each day, daily, every day
q 6 hr, q6h, q6hr	every 6 hours
BID	2 times a day
TID	3 times a day
QID, qid	4 times a day
QOD	every other day
QHS, qhs	at bedtime
PO	orally, by mouth
sl, SL	under the tongue, sublingually
IV	intravenously
SC, SQ	subcutaneously
IM	intramuscularly
PRN, prn	as needed, as circumstances require
c̄	with
s̄	without

Fig. 24.4 Abbreviations used in writing prescriptions.

For example:
- CHLORDIAZEPOXIDE 25 MG PO TID: 25 mg of chlordiazepoxide by mouth 3 times per day.
- GENTAMICIN 100 MG IV Q 12′: 100 mg of gentamicin intravenously every 12 hours.
- ACETAMINOPHEN 325 MG 2 TABS PO q 4–6′ PRN PAIN: two 325 mg tablets of acetaminophen every 4 to 6 hours as needed for pain.
- NPH INSULIN 30U SQ qAM AND 20U SQ qPM: give the patient 30 units of insulin subcutaneously each morning and 20 units each evening.

Try and get into the habit of using generic names only.

Important note: If you are uncertain about what strength or dosage form a medication comes in, *do not guess!* Either look it up, or call the pharmacy. It saves time and frustration in the long run. There are many pocket references as well as PDA programs that you can use.

Outpatient prescriptions

For an outpatient prescription, you include all of the above information on a prescription blank, plus the total amount of medication that you want the pharmacist to dispense (written as "dispense #") and the number of refills. It is relatively common to give patients a one-month supply of drug. *All* controlled substances (i.e., narcotics) require a physician's DEA number or hospital DEA number.

For example:
- Rx: AMOXICILLIN 250 MG, #40 (forty) [don't forget to write out the number of pills]
  sig: 1 tab po bid ×10 days—for airway infection.
- Rx: AMITRIPTYLINE 150 MG #14 (fourteen)
  sig: 1 po qhs—for depression

For the patient's benefit, it is useful to write the reason for the medication in lay terms as part of the instructions, i.e., "for airway infection" in the first example above and "for depression" in the second example. This is especially helpful for patients who take multiple medications.

25. Oral Case Presentations

Overview

Case presentation is an important skill for the student to develop. By this means one can convey a clear, comprehensive account of the patient's medical problems to others. In order to do this effectively, one must know the data and present it in an organized fashion in a professional way.

Settings for oral case presentations

Presentations, like write-ups, should follow the SOAP format. The extensiveness of the presentation should suit the circumstances. There are three main types of presentations to consider; most other situations will be variations of the three.

Inpatient presentations (formal case or morning rounds)

- The hospitalized patient represents the opportunity for a complete history and physical exam.
- The operating assumption is that this patient may never be seen again, so all medical issues need to be considered.
- This is obviously a lengthy process since all aspects of the history of present illness, past medical history, review of systems, and healthcare maintenance issues must be followed out to the end.
- While painful for the student, the patient, and the attending, this type of presentation is important to establish a baseline of data that subsequent visits or presentations can be weighed against.
- When the student can perform this presentation seamlessly, all other presentations will seem virtually effortless.
- The student in his or her mind always compares subsequent efforts to this ideal and is therefore aware of what is left out.
- A good, complete presentation may take from about 10 to 40 minutes.

Outpatient presentations

- If the patient has been seen before, only the relevant clinical information should be presented.
- Focus on the major health problems and how the patient is doing: is the patient better, worse, or about the same?
- Relevant history should be offered as well to demonstrate that you understand the context of that day's visit.
- The busier the clinic day, the less likely that you will consider healthcare maintenance; however, be sure to think about relevant issues such as flu or pneumonia immunizations for patients with cardiac or pulmonary problems.
- Always consider what you are leaving out, and note what needs to be followed up at the next visit.
- Plan for about 5–10 minutes to complete the presentation.

Specialty presentations

- You will frequently have to call a specialist with questions about a particular patient or diagnosis.
- There are two important points to consider: what is the question that you want the specialist to answer, and what information does the specialist need in order to answer the question?
- You need to be able to give all of the relevant information, but no more. This is often not easy to do.
- Usually the specialist will be able to prompt you about the information that you have not provided; you should be prepared to elaborate.
- Work toward a 3- to 5-minute presentation.

General guidelines

Medical reporting should be a short, fast-moving account of what has happened to the patient. Properly delivered, it will stimulate the listener to construct his or her own differential diagnosis as the story unfolds. By including pertinent positive and negative features of the history and physical examination, one can develop the main diagnostic points.

217

Opening statement

The opening statement, which includes the "chief complaint," should catch the listener's attention. A verbatim report of the patient's reason for seeking medical attention should *not* be used.

- You should state the real reason as you see it, based on your appraisal of the problem. For example, say, "This 60-year-old stockbroker was seen because of weakness and a 15 lb weight loss," not "He is tired and doesn't feel well."
- You (or your attending) might prefer including major known past diagnoses. For example, "This 60-year-old male stockbroker with known carcinoma of the lung since 1988 complains of weakness and a 15 lb weight loss over the past month."
- Some physicians feel that inclusion of the patient's occupation and marital status gives a better feeling for the patient.
- Details such as drinking and smoking habits, financial problems, and job and marital stresses should be included elsewhere, not in the opening statement, unless they are directly related to the likely diagnosis.
- You should include a brief statement as to the source and reliability of your information. For several reasons a patient may not be a reliable informant: dementia, language barrier, low intelligence, and obtundation from disease or medications affect the patient's ability to give accurate information. Information obtained from relatives, friends, other physicians, and medical records should be noted.

Description of the chief complaint should include the following points:

- Was the onset acute or insidious?
- Was the intensity mild, moderate, or severe?
- Is it progressing or diminishing in its severity?
- Has the course of the illness been steady or intermittent, rapid or slow?
- What factors have aggravated or relieved the chief complaint?
- What degree of disability has resulted from the illness?

Description of pertinent symptoms

After describing the chief complaint, you should comment upon pertinent associated symptoms and their time relationship to the main problem. It is important to keep track of all the symptoms, indicating whether they have persisted, worsened, or disappeared.

Differential diagnosis

At this point in the history you should consider the differential diagnosis raised thus far in deciding which features to emphasize in support of your own diagnosis.

- This includes a past history of predisposing or etiological factors and the presence or absence of diseases often associated with the primary complaint or complications thereof.
- For example, in dealing with a patient with severe chest pain, you might mention previous angina or myocardial infarction, the presence or absence of hypertension, diabetes, familial history of coronary disease, excessive smoking, and hyperlipidemia.
- You also would want to mention whether there were any symptoms of congestive heart failure or cardiac dysrhythmias.
- If related, either positively or negatively, parts of the social history and review of systems should be presented here.

Description of physical findings

The description of the physical findings should be abbreviated, emphasizing the features raised by the differential diagnosis.

General description of the patient

Begin by giving a brief general description of the patient, including physical appearance and mental status.

Vital signs

List the vital signs. In a disease not associated with consistent deviation from normal, one might say, "The vital signs were normal."

Noncontributory findings

You should comment on noncontributory findings and cover unrelated areas with the terms "normal" or "unremarkable." For example, if you are discussing a patient with a history of recurrent diverticulitis and no other medical problems, you might say, "The head, neck, heart, and lungs were normal."

Specific system-related findings

Then you may spend time on describing the examination of the abdomen and rectum. Significant

---

Formal case presentation

Mr. Platz is a 62-year-old man presenting because of fever and cough for 2 days. He was well until 10 days ago, when he developed nasal congestion, sore throat, and low-grade fever. These seemed to improve until 2 days ago, when he noted fever to 103°, cough productive of green sputum, and shortness of breath while climbing stairs.

He reports diffuse muscle aches and mild nausea but denies shaking chills, chest pain, headache, stiff neck, or abdominal pain. There is no recent travel, no bird exposure, and no TB exposure. He reports chronic cough productive of about a teaspoon of yellow sputum in the morning for several years but no history of lung disease, asthma, dyspnea, asbestos exposure, or hemoptysis.

The past medical history is significant for an MI 3 years ago without complication or subsequent chest pain. Medications include diltiazem-CD 180 mg QD and aspirin prn. There are no known drug allergies. He has smoked 1ppd for 40 years and drinks 2 beers per day. There are no known HIV risk factors.

He works as a banana importer and is married with two children. There is no history of unusual travel. Family history is notable for a stroke in his father and Lyme disease in his sister.

The review of systems is notable for a 20 lb weight loss over 6 months without dieting.
Negative findings include:
- There are no fevers, sweats, or lymphadenopathy.
- He denies head trauma, headache, or dizziness.
- He denies visual difficulty, pain, glaucoma, or cataract.
- There is no auditory difficulty, pain, or tinnitus.
- There is no nasal discharge, breathing difficulty, sinus symptoms, or epistaxis.
- There are no dental problems, gum bleeding, sores, or change in taste.
- He denies voice change, difficulty swallowing, or neck pain.
- He denies chest pain, dyspnea, orthopnea, PND, palpitations, murmur, or rheumatic fever.
- There is no abdominal pain, nausea, vomiting, liver disease, gallbladder disease, pancreatic disease, diarrhea, constipation, change in bowel habits, rectal bleeding, or food intolerance.
- He denies kidney disease, dysuria, hematuria, nocturia, or urinary tract infections.
- He reports nocturia once nightly but denies hesitancy, dribbling, penile discharge, sexual difficulties, sexually transmitted disease, or scrotal or testicular mass.
- There is no back pain or disk disease.
- He denies joint pain, stiffness, or swelling.

Fig. 25.1 Example of formal case presentation.

Continued

negatives should be mentioned, specifically with respect to the area of interest. If, for example, the patient has an anginal syndrome:

- You should give the pulse rate and blood pressure, even though they are normal.
- Respirations may be described as normal unless there are reasons to suspect heart failure.
- The carotid and jugular/venous pulses should be mentioned specifically, even if they are normal.
- Findings in the lungs should be mentioned, and the heart should be described in detail, stating rate, rhythm, size, heart sounds, murmurs, and friction rubs.
- Mention of the peripheral arterial pulses and the presence or absence of edema finishes the more important points.

Disagreement among observers

When there is a disagreement among several observers about a particular physical finding, you can say, "One observer noted..." to describe the finding in question. This eliminates the need for detailed and distracting accounts of who found what and who disagreed.

Laboratory findings

Laboratory findings, if available, should be presented in the following order: routine blood counts, urinalysis, blood chemistries, imaging studies, electrocardiograms, and special procedures.

Course of illness and treatment

A brief comment on the course of the illness and the treatment, including all medications, should be made. Specific changes in symptoms, physical findings, and laboratory studies must be mentioned.

Length of presentation

While a formal case presentation (Fig. 25.1) may take longer than 10 minutes, a presentation on

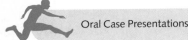

Formal case presentation (*Continued*)

- He denies edema, pain, phlebitis, varicosities, or claudication.
- He denies rash, skin growths, itching, easy bruising, change in moles, or change in skin texture.
- He denies headache, dizziness, seizure, motor or sensory disturbance, or bowel or bladder dysfunction.

General physical examination. The patient was mildly ill-appearing and in moderate respiratory distress. Temperature was 39.7° tympanic with BP 150/94, HR 104, RR 28.

The head was normal. The extraocular structures were intact. The conjunctivae were mildly injected without discharge. The sclera were clear. Optic disks were flat, and the fundi had mild arteriolar narrowing but no AV nicking, exudates, or hemorrhages.

The pinnae, auditory canals, and tympanic membranes were normal. The external nasal structures and nares were normal. The oropharynx demonstrated good dentition with no lesions of the buccal mucosa, gums, or pharynx.

The neck was supple without bruit. The thyroid was normal.

There were no palpable lymph nodes.

Examination of the chest revealed coarse crackles in the right lower field with E to A changes but no dullness.

There was no JVD. The carotid upstrokes were normal. The apical impulse was palpable in the left fifth intercostal space, midclavicular line. S_1 and S_2 were normal. There was no murmur, gallop, or rub. Pulses were normal.

The abdomen had normal active bowel sounds and was soft and nontender. The liver was 12 cm by percussion and was smooth, firm, and nontender. The spleen was not palpable. There were no masses and no hernia.

The penis and testes were normal.

The rectal exam showed normal tone without mass. The prostate was mildly enlarged but had no nodule or asymmetry. The stool was brown and *guaiac-positive* for occult blood.

The back was symmetric and nontender. The skin had no abnormal findings. The extremities had no cyanosis, clubbing, or edema.

On neurologic exam, the patient was alert and oriented X 3. Higher intellectual function was normal. Cranial nerves II–XII were normal. Strength and tone were normal. Sensation was intact to pin, temperature, vibration, and proprioception. Rapid alternating motion was normal. The gait was normal. Deep tendon reflexes were 2/4 throughout. The plantar reflexes were downgoing.

Lab studies were notable for WBC 16.8 with 84% polys, 6% bands, and 10% lymphs. Chest x-ray demonstrates right lower lobe infiltrate. Sputum Gram stain revealed numerous polys and numerous Gram-positive cocci in clusters.

In summary, Mr. Platz is a 62-year-old man with a history of MI and smoking who presents with fever and cough for 2 days. Review of systems is remarkable for involuntary 20 lb weight loss, for chronic productive cough, and for mild nocturia. The exam is notable for temperature 39.7°, HR 104, RR 28, moderate respiratory distress, and rhonchi with egophony in the right lower field. Guaiac-positive stool and mild prostatic enlargement are also noted. Labs are notable for WBC 16.8 with left shift. Chest x-ray demonstrates RLL infiltrate, and sputum Gram stain reveals Gram-positive cocci in clusters.

Fig. 25.1 *Continued*

---

morning rounds (Fig. 25.2) should be completed in approximately 7 to 10 minutes. The more complex the account, the more you should compress the description of secondary problems. For example, if you must detail the evolution of a longstanding case of diabetes, you might settle for the brief statement, "He also has chronic obstructive pulmonary disease and a quiescent duodenal ulcer." An outpatient presentation (Fig. 25.3) should be completed in less than 5 minutes.

Summary

Finally, summarize the entire picture in a few sentences, including the differential diagnosis and the working diagnosis. For example:

"A 58-year-old male electrician gives a history of an increasingly severe retrosternal chest pain over the past 3 weeks. An impending myocardial infarction seems to be the best bet. Other possibilities include pericarditis, esophageal pain, and chest wall pain. There is a strong family history of coronary disease, and the patient has been a heavy cigarette smoker for over 20 years. There is no evidence of hypertension, heart failure, or cardiac dysrhythmia."

Presentation on morning rounds

The setting for presentation on morning rounds is related to work. The house staff, students, and teaching faculty are gathered to review admissions from the previous day. The purpose of a morning rounds presentation is to transmit clinical information. By the end of your presentation, the other members of the team should know everything about the patient that might be pertinent to his or her care. Its duration is ≤5 minutes, and the style is concise.

The presentation is formatted to meet these ends. The chief complaint, history of the present illness, and past medical history are reported as in the formal case presentation, stressing conciseness. The social history, family history, and review of systems are reduced to noteworthy findings only. The physical exam describes the neck, lymph nodes, respiratory, cardiac, abdomen, rectal, and extremity exams in full. Other organ systems are described only if abnormal. Lab results and summary are described as in the formal exam.

Mr. Platz is a 62-year-old man presenting because of fever and cough for 2 days. He was well until 10 days ago, when he developed nasal congestion, sore throat, and low-grade fever. These symptoms seemed to improve until 2 days ago, when he noted fever to 103°, cough productive of green sputum, and shortness of breath while climbing stairs.

He reports diffuse muscle aches and mild nausea but denies shaking chills, chest pain, headache, stiff neck, or abdominal pain. There is no recent travel, no bird exposure, and no TB exposure. He reports chronic cough productive of about a teaspoon of yellow sputum in the morning for several years but no history of lung disease, asthma, dyspnea, asbestos exposure, or hemoptysis.

The past medical history is significant for an MI 3 years ago without complication or subsequent chest pain. Medications include diltiazem-CD 180 mg QD and aspirin prn. There are no known drug allergies. He has smoked 1ppd for 40 years and drinks 2 beers per day. There are no known HIV risk factors.

He works as a banana importer and is married with two children. There is no history of unusual travel. Family history is notable for a stroke in his father.

The review of systems is notable for a 20 lb weight loss over 6 months without dieting.
Negative findings include:
- There are no fevers, sweats, or lymphadenopathy.
- He denies chest pain, dyspnea, orthopnea, PND, palpitations, murmur, or rheumatic fever.
- There is no abdominal pain, nausea, vomiting, liver disease, gallbladder disease, pancreatic disease, diarrhea, constipation, change in bowel habits, rectal bleeding, or food intolerance.
- He denies kidney disease, dysuria, hematuria, nocturia, or urinary tract infections.
- He reports nocturia once nightly but denies hesitancy, dribbling, penile discharge, sexual difficulties, sexually transmitted disease, or scrotal or testicular mass.

Physical examination. The patient was mildly ill-appearing and in moderate respiratory distress. Temperature was 39.7° tympanic with BP 150/94, HR 104, RR 28.

The head was normal. The eyes were normal except for mild arteriolar narrowing. The ears, nose, and mouth were normal. The neck was supple without bruit. The thyroid was normal.

There were no palpable lymph nodes.

The chest had coarse crackles in the right lower field with E to A changes but no dullness.

There was no JVD. The carotid upstrokes were normal. The apical impulse was palpable in the left fifth intercostal space, midclavicular line. S_1 and S_2 were normal. There was no murmur, gallop, or rub. Pulses were normal.

The abdomen had normal active bowel sounds and was soft and nontender. The liver was 12 cm by percussion and was smooth, firm, and nontender. The spleen was not palpable. There were no masses and no hernia.

The penis and testes were normal.

The rectal exam showed normal tone without mass. The prostate was mildly enlarged but had no nodule or asymmetry. The stool was brown and *guaiac-positive* for occult blood.

The back, skin, and extremities were normal.

On neurologic exam, the patient was alert and oriented X 3. Higher intellectual function was normal. Cranial nerves II–XII were normal. Strength and tone were normal. Sensation was intact to pin, temperature, vibration, and proprioception. Rapid alternating motion was normal. The gait was normal. Deep tendon reflexes were 2/4 throughout. The plantar reflexes were downgoing.

Lab studies were notable for WBC 16.8 and 84% polys, 6% bands, and 10% lymphs. Chest x-ray demonstrates right lower lobe infiltrate. Sputum Gram stain revealed numerous polys and numerous Gram-positive cocci in clusters.

In summary, Mr. Platz is a 62-year-old man with a history of MI and smoking who presents with fever and cough for 2 days. Review of systems is remarkable for involuntary 20 lb weight loss, for chronic productive cough, and for mild nocturia. The exam is notable for temperature 39.7°, HR 104, RR 28, moderate respiratory distress, and rhonchi with egophony in the right lower field. Guaiac-positive stool and mild prostatic enlargement are also noted. Labs are notable for WBC 16.8 with left shift. Chest x-ray demonstrates RLL infiltrate, and sputum Gram stain reveals Gram-positive cocci in clusters.

Fig. 25.2 Example of presentation on morning rounds.

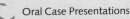

Outpatient presentation

Mr. McMillan is a 72-year-old man who comes to the office for follow-up after a recent hospitalization. He had been admitted because of fever, cough, and dyspnea. PMH notable for uncomplicated MI 2 years ago, a chronic cough, and a 60 pack year history of smoking (although he stopped 8 years ago). While in the hospital, he was found to have a RLL pneumonia and was treated with ceftriaxone and erythromycin. Today is he doing well. Of note, he has had a 20 lb weight loss in the past 3 months, and there was concern that his chest x-ray demonstrated a postobstructive consolidation. I'm concerned that he may have a malignancy and would like to get a chest CT scan.

Fig. 25.3 Example of outpatient presentation.

Additional suggestions

- Bedside presentation must not in any way embarrass or compromise the dignity of the patient.
- Show how much work you have put into the study and evaluation of the patient's problem by being organized and prepared to discuss the assessment and plans.
- Have a note card available for reference.
- Rehearse your presentation before giving it, especially for formal conferences.
- The use of abbreviations such as SOB, TB, CA, VD, etc., has no place in the presentation.

26. Further Investigations

Overview

Once the history and examination have been performed, it is necessary to assess your differential diagnosis and to plan a management strategy for the patient. Part of this process includes arranging further investigations in order to refine the differential diagnosis. The tests may be performed to:

- Exclude serious conditions.
- Confirm the presence of a suspected pathology.
- Obtain a baseline against which further progress may be assessed.
- Assess the severity of the current illness.
- Assess the response to therapy.
- Predict prognosis.

 Before requesting any investigations, think how the patient will benefit from the result.

Remember that it is easy to request investigations, but the results may require great skill in interpretation. Furthermore, each test has a cost and produces a defined morbidity (however small) to the patient. It is essential to anticipate how the results of the investigation may alter your management at the time of the request. If you cannot see how the results of an investigation will alter your management, there is absolutely no point requesting that test. For each test, be prepared to justify:

- Why it is being requested.
- How the result will affect management.
- That the potential benefit of the information outweighs the cost and morbidity incurred.
- The urgency of a request.

The lists given below are not intended to be comprehensive and certainly do not imply that every test should be requested for each system. The tests requested need to be tailored to the clinical scenario. For each system, consider:

- Urine.
- Blood.
- Radiological imaging.
- Electrical recording.
- Special investigations.

Cardiovascular system

The diagnosis of acute MI is made on the basis of two of the following three factors being present: chest pain, ECG changes consistent with MI, and an increase in cardiac enzymes.

Blood tests

The following blood tests may help in the diagnosis of cardiac pathologies:

- Complete blood count. Anemia may be the cause of or exacerbate heart failure or angina.
- Erythrocyte sedimentation rate (ESR). Inflammatory conditions (e.g., endocarditis) are associated with a raised ESR. The C-reactive protein (CRP) is an acute-phase protein and is often more sensitive in changing inflammatory states (e.g., monitoring the response of infective endocarditis to antibiotic therapy).
- Cardiac enzymes. Tropinin T is released by cardiac muscle breakdown. It should be measured 12 hours after chest pain or a change in rhythm.
- Biochemical profile. Exclude electrolyte disturbance as a cause of arrhythmia.
- Thyroid function tests. Hyperthyroidism is a common cause of atrial fibrillation. Hypothyroidism may present as a pleural effusion or heart failure.
- Blood cultures. Essential if endocarditis is suspected.

223

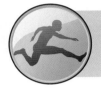

If infective endocarditis is suspected, obtain at least six sets of blood cultures.

Urinalysis

Look for microscopic hematuria if infective endocarditis is suspected.

Imaging
Chest radiography

A chest radiograph is usually requested for a patient who presents with cardiological symptoms. Note the presence of:

- Cardiac enlargement: cardiothoracic ratio should be less than 50% (posteroanterior film).
- Signs of increased left atrial filling pressure: upper lobe blood diversion, septal lines, pulmonary edema, pleural effusion (Fig. 26.1).
- Signs of left atrial enlargement: prominence of atrial appendage (straight left heart border), double contour of right heart border, splaying of the carina.
- Left ventricular aneurysm: post-myocardial infarction.
- Abnormal calcification: valvular calcification in rheumatic heart disease, tuberculous pericardial disease (Fig. 26.2).

Echocardiography

Echocardiography may be transthoracic (noninvasive) or transesophageal, which provides better images of the left atrium and aorta. It is useful for assessing chamber size, valvular pathology, pericardial disease, and contractility of the heart. Echocardiography is usually requested to:

- Investigate heart murmurs.
- Look for vegetations in suspected infective endocarditis.
- Investigate pericardial effusions and tamponade.
- Assess the severity of cor pulmonale.
- Investigate aortic aneurysms.

Modifications of echocardiography such as stress echo and contrast echo may also be used to investigate angina and septal defects, respectively. The two most common views are illustrated in Figs. 26.3 and 26.4.

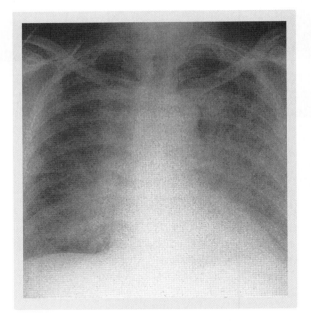

Fig. 26.1 Radiograph of left heart failure. Note the cardiomegaly, bilateral alveolar shadowing in a perihilar distribution, and the presence of fluid in the horizontal fissure.

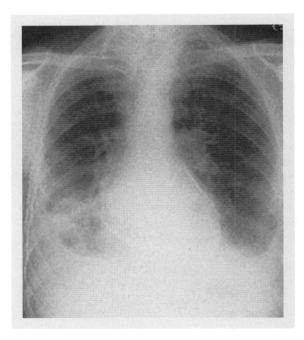

Fig. 26.2 Radiograph of pericardial calcification. Note the associated pleural effusions.

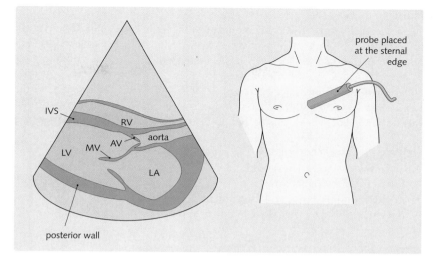

Fig. 26.3 Diagrammatic representation of an echocardiogram of a normal long-axis view of the left ventricle. The probe is placed in the left parasternal region. This provides a good view for assessing chamber size, left ventricular wall motion, and ejection fraction as well as mitral and aortic valve regurgitation using color Doppler. AV, aortic valve; IVS, interventricular septum; LA, left atrium; LV, left ventricle; MV, mitral valve; RV, right ventricle.

Fig. 26.4 Diagrammatic echocardiogram representation of a four-chamber view. The probe is placed at the apex. This view allows assessment of the left ventricular apex and quantification of the severity of aortic and tricuspid valve pathology. LA, left atrium; LV, left ventricle; RA, right atrium; RV, right ventricle.

Nuclear imaging
Nuclear imaging (e.g., thallium scan) can be used to investigate suspected angina in a patient who cannot perform an exercise test.

Electrocardiography (ECG)
12-lead ECG
ECGs are very widely performed. They can be used to assess rhythm disturbances, ischemia or infarction, left ventricular hypertrophy, right ventricular hypertrophy; a useful ECG resource can be found at medstat.med.utah.edu/kw/ecg.

24-hour tape (Holter monitor)
A 24-hour tape is used to investigate paroxysmal cardiac arrhythmias that may be associated with symptoms. Patients should be instructed to indicate when they have palpitations or other symptoms such as lightheadedness so that their symptoms can be correlated with electrical disturbances.

Event recorder (cardiac memo)
If the palpitation lasts long enough, it is desirable to record the ECG at the time of the arrhythmia. Symptoms can then be directly related to the electrical activity of the heart.

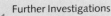

Exercise ECG

The exercise ECG is used as a screening test in the investigation of ischemia. Many cardiologists do not refer patients for angiography if the exercise test is normal. In addition, exercise testing provides collateral information about exercise tolerance. Remember that it is a waste of time requesting an exercise test for a wheelchair-bound 90-year-old!

Coronary angiography

This invasive investigation is used:

- To assess the coronary arteries.
- To measure pressures in the heart chambers in the assessment of valve pathology or cor pulmonale.

Respiratory system

Blood tests

Patients with respiratory disease often have infections or unexplained dyspnea. The more commonly requested blood tests include:

- Complete blood count. A raised white cell count suggests infection. A raised eosinophil count may occur in rare conditions.
- You can check the C-reactive protein as a nonspecific marker of inflammation. As the disease state resolves, the level should drop.
- Blood cultures: important in the diagnosis of pneumonia.
- Arterial blood gases: essential in the assessment of severe asthma attacks and for providing baseline function for patients with chronic obstructive pulmonary disease (COPD).

Sputum assessment

Sputum culture is part of the routine assessment of a patient with a chest infection. When investigating pneumonia, especially in sick patients, liaison with the laboratory is important for diagnosing some of the less common infections (e.g., *Pneumocystis*, mycobacteria, *Nocardia*).

Sputum cytology is used in the investigation of malignancy and certain pneumonias.

Imaging
Chest radiography

In the context of respiratory disease, the important features to note are:

- Area of consolidation: for example, lobar or widespread.

- Evidence of COPD: paucity of lung vascular markings, hyperinflation, flat diaphragms, narrow mediastinum, bullae.
- Pneumothorax or areas of collapse in asthmatic patients.
- Hilar masses: lung carcinoma may underlie many respiratory disorders (Fig. 26.5); bilateral lymphadenopathy occurs in sarcoidosis.
- Pleural effusions.
- Fibrosis.

Computerized tomography (CT) scan

Occasionally, CT scanning is needed to clarify features on the radiograph. For example:

- Investigation of direct or metastatic spread of suspected lung cancer.
- Investigation of bronchiectasis.
- Investigation of pulmonary fibrosis.

Lung function tests

Assessment of gas exchange and airway function may be performed by the following methods.

Peak expiratory flow rate

This should be considered as part of the routine examination of the asthmatic patient.

Arterial blood gases

These are useful for assessing gas exchange in acute pulmonary disease. In addition they provide a

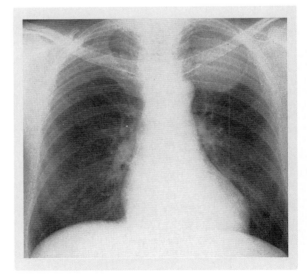

Fig. 26.5 Radiograph of a Pancoast tumor with destruction of the first left rib.

baseline assessment for patients with COPD when they are stable (e.g., 3 months after any infective exacerbation).

Spirometry

The simplest assessments of forced expiratory volume in 1 second (FEV_1) and forced vital capacity (FVC) can provide invaluable information in respiratory disease. The ratio of FEV_1/FVC and absolute values will help in the diagnosis of:

- Obstructive disease: low ratio (<70%) and low absolute values.
- Restrictive disease: normal or high ratio, reduced FVC (Fig. 26.6).

In addition, the absolute value of FEV_1 is often used to assess patients with respiratory muscle weakness (e.g., myasthenia gravis, Guillain–Barré syndrome).

Variations can be used to record bronchial reactivity to allergens or potential reversibility with bronchodilators.

The transfer coefficient of carbon monoxide (K_{CO}) provides a measure of the efficiency of gas exchange and permeability of the alveolar membrane:

- Diseases resulting in impaired ventilation or perfusion reduce K_{CO}.
- Diseases such as pulmonary hemorrhage increase K_{CO}.

Bronchoscopy

Bronchoscopy allows direct visualization of the upper airways, and abnormal areas can be biopsied. In addition, bronchoalveolar lavage can be performed to collect specimens for culture and cytology and to assess the differential cell types in the alveoli.

Abdominal system

Blood tests

Blood tests are required for a wide range of abdominal presentations, including the investigation of anemia, jaundice, palpable masses, abdominal pain, and bowel disturbance.

The more commonly requested investigations include:

- Complete blood count. This may reveal anemia. The mean cell volume (MCV) provides a starting point for further investigation. A raised white count suggests an inflammatory process.
- ESR. Raises the suspicion of inflammatory lesions.
- Biochemical profile. Assesses liver function, renal function, and calcium. Electrolyte levels may fluctuate during diarrheal illnesses or fluid replacement.
- Vitamin B_{12}, iron studies, red cell folate levels. These are initial investigations in anemia.
- Amylase and lipase. Exclude pancreatitis as a cause of abdominal pain.

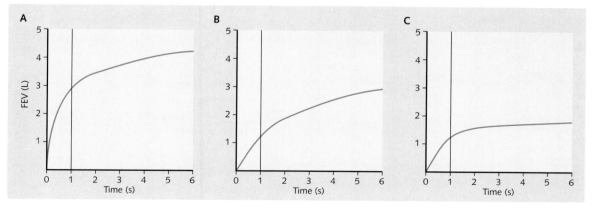

Fig. 26.6 Examples of spirometry. (A) Normal patient: FEV_1/FVC = 3.0/4.0 (75%). (B) COPD: FEV_1/FVC = 1.5/3.0 (50%). (C) Fibrosis: FEV_1/FVC = 1.5/1.8 (83%).

Urinalysis

Urinalysis is part of the routine assessment during a detailed examination. Note the presence of:

- Glycosuria: diabetes mellitus.
- Hematuria: for example, due to glomerulonephritis, renal stone, bladder lesion.
- Proteinuria.
- Ketonuria: diabetic ketoacidosis.
- Nitrites or leukocytes: indicate infection.

Imaging
Chest radiography

An erect chest radiograph is often requested for patients presenting with acute abdominal pain. The important features to note are:

- The presence of free air under the diaphragm: suggests perforated viscus (Fig. 26.7).
- Lower lobe consolidation: pneumonia masquerading as acute abdominal pain.

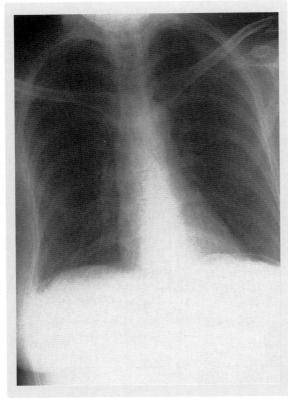

Fig. 26.7 Air under the diaphragm. This suggests the presence of a perforated abdominal viscus.

Abdominal radiography

The main features to note are:

- Distended loops of bowel: suggestive of bowel obstruction.
- Double contour to the bowel: perforation with free air in the abdomen (Wriggler's sign).
- Radiopaque gallstones: unusual (only 10%).
- Radiopaque renal calculi: common (90%).

Abdominal ultrasound and CT scan

These are performed to localize and identify any abnormal masses, detect free fluid in the abdomen, and assess the size and parenchyma of intra-abdominal organs.

Ultrasound is particularly useful in the assessment of jaundice as biliary tree dilatation and gallstones are readily identified.

Following trauma, CT or ultrasound may be used to diagnose damage to the liver, kidney, or spleen.

Barium studies

Barium studies are used to assess abnormalities of the mucosa or motility disorders. The four main studies are:

- Barium swallow: to assess the esophagus (e.g., for dysphagia, heartburn).
- Upper GI: to assess mucosal abnormalities of the stomach and duodenum (e.g., for dyspepsia, iron deficiency anemia).
- Upper GI with small bowel follow-through: to assess the small bowel, in particular the terminal ileum (e.g., for malabsorption, suspected Crohn's disease).
- Barium enema: to investigate the colon (e.g., for anemia, change in bowel habit, rectal bleeding).

Endoscopy

Endoscopy is performed to visualize the mucosa of the bowel directly and to biopsy any abnormal area. Upper gastrointestinal (GI) endoscopy will assess as far as the duodenum. A good colonoscopy will reveal the whole of the large bowel.

Endoscopic retrograde cholangiopancreatography (ERCP) can be performed to image the pancreatic or hepatic and bile ducts and to treat any strictures or remove stones.

Stool assessment

Stool assessment may involve:

- Culture: for diarrheal illnesses.
- Microscopy: for ova cysts and parasites.
- Fecal fat estimation.

Neurological system

Imaging

CT scans and magnetic resonance imaging (MRI) of the brain or spinal cord are often requested to investigate acute and chronic neurological symptoms. CT is the modality of choice in the investigation of acute trauma or subarachnoid hemorrhage.

Electroencephalography (EEG)

The EEG relates to the brain in the same way that the ECG relates to the heart. However, correlation between the traces and physiological function is less understood. The main uses of the EEG are in:

- Diagnosis of epilepsy.
- Diagnosis of encephalitis.

Lumbar puncture

Lumbar puncture provides essential information in the assessment of patients with neurological disease, especially those with suspected meningitis. The main indications are:

- Investigation of meningitis.
- Pyrexia of unknown origin.
- Subarachnoid hemorrhage.
- Inflammatory central nervous system (CNS) disease (e.g., multiple sclerosis, vasculitis).

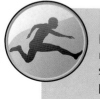

In the presence of decreased level of consciousness or focal neurological sign, obtain a CT scan of the brain before performing a lumbar puncture.

Lumbar puncture is contraindicated in the presence of:

- Suppuration of the skin overlying the spinal canal.
- Undiagnosed papilledema.

Electromyography (EMG)

EMG is used in the assessment of the peripheral nervous system. It is particularly useful if the patient reports:

- Weakness or wasting.
- Undue fatiguability.
- Sensory impairment or paresthesia.

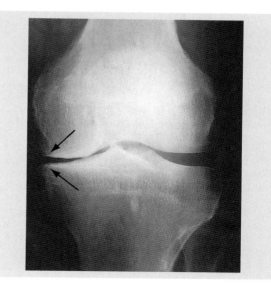

Fig. 26.8 X-ray of knee showing osteoarthritic changes. Note the loss of joint space, bone sclerosis, osteophytes, and subchondral cysts.

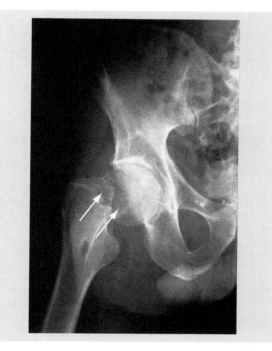

Fig. 26.9 X-ray showing a fractured neck of femur.

EMG will establish a diagnosis of a neuropathy and identify the pathological process as a demyelination or axonal neuropathy. In addition, diagnostic information may be provided for some myopathies.

Evoked potentials

Visual evoked potentials are sometimes used in the assessment of a patient with suspected multiple sclerosis.

Musculoskeletal system

X-rays are the usual investigation in the diagnosis of muscular and joint problems. Figures 26.8 and 26.9 show the changes associated with osteoarthritis in the knee and hip, respectively.

Recommended Childhood and Adolescent Immunization Schedule UNITED STATES • 2005

Vaccine ▼ / Age ▶	Birth	1 month	2 months	4 months	6 months	12 months	15 months	18 months	24 months	4-6 years	11-12 years	13-18 years
Hepatitis B	HepB #1	HepB #2			HepB #3						HepB Series	
Diphtheria, Tetanus, Pertussis			DTaP	DTaP	DTaP		DTaP			DTaP	Td	Td
Haemophilus influenzae type b			Hib	Hib	Hib	Hib						
Inactivated Poliovirus			IPV	IPV	IPV					IPV		
Measles, Mumps, Rubella						MMR #1				MMR #2	MMR #2	
Varicella						Varicella				Varicella		
Pneumococcal			PCV	PCV	PCV	PCV			PCV	PPV		
Influenza					Influenza (Yearly)					Influenza (Yearly)		
Hepatitis A										Hepatitis A Series		

Vaccines below red line are for selected populations

Legend:
- Range of recommended ages
- Preadolescent assessment
- Only if mother HBsAg(−)
- Catch-up immunization

This schedule indicates the recommended ages for routine administration of currently licensed childhood vaccines, as of December 1, 2004, for children through age 18 years. Any dose not given at the recommended age should be given at any subsequent visit when indicated and feasible. █ Indicates age groups that warrant special effort to administer those vaccines not previously given. Additional vaccines may be licensed and recommended during the year. Licensed combination vaccines may be used whenever any components of the combination are indicated and the vaccine's other components are not contraindicated. Providers should consult the manufacturers' package inserts for detailed recommendations. Clinically significant adverse events that follow immunization should be reported to the Vaccine Adverse Event Reporting System (VAERS). Guidance about how to obtain and complete a VAERS form can be found on the Internet: www.vaers.org or by calling 800-822-7967.

The Childhood and Adolescent Immunization Schedule is approved by:
Advisory Committee on Immunization Practices www.cdc.gov/nip/acip
American Academy of Pediatrics www.aap.org
American Academy of Family Physicians www.aafp.org

DEPARTMENT OF HEALTH AND HUMAN SERVICES
CENTERS FOR DISEASE CONTROL AND PREVENTION

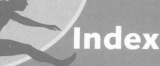

Index

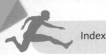

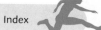

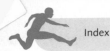

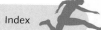

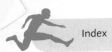

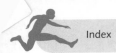

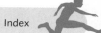

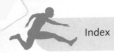

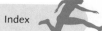

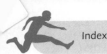

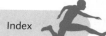

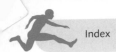

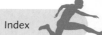

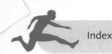

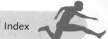

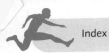